UNLOCKING
EDEN

★ ★ ★ ★ ★

"Shatters the Paradigm!"

— Dr. Ralph Umbriaco D.C., MsTOM, C.N.H.P

UNLOCKING
EDEN

Revolutionize Your Health,
Maximize Your Immunity,
Restore Your Vitality

JOE HORN
&
DANIEL BELT

DEFENDER

CRANE, MO

UNLOCKING EDEN: Revolutionize Your Health, Maximize Your Immunity, Restore Your Vitality
by Joe Horn and Daniel Belt

Defender Publishing
Crane, MO 65633
© 2020 Joe Horn and Daniel Belt
All Rights Reserved. Published 2020.
Printed in the United States of America.

ISBN 978-1-948014-35-951995

A CIP catalog record of this book is available from the Library of Congress.

Cover design by Jeffrey Mardis.

All Scripture from the King James Version.

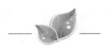

This book is dedicated to God, through whom all things are possible! Also, to my loving wife, who has carried me through so much; to my incredible children; and to future generations who will inherit the world we leave behind.

~ Joe Horn

This book is first dedicated to my mother, who lives a selfless love. Further, this book is also dedicated to all of humanity; may peace be with you.

~ Daniel Belt

CONTENTS

Note to the Reader

The phrase "CAM (Complementary and Alternative Medicine) Therapy" is a blanket term used to address any type of medical practice found outside the realm of traditional, modern, American medical practice. This can include (but is not limited to) qualified professionals in such arenas as: acupuncture, osteopathic, or chiropractic practices; holistic medicine; homeopathic medicine; naturopathic practices; massage therapy; physical therapy; and more. Throughout this book, we will be using the phrase "natural healthcare practitioner" to refer to any and all natural or alternative medicine providers. Readers are encouraged to use their own discretion when properly vetting the knowledge, skills, education, and qualification of these providers. The statements made in this book are in no way intended to be used as a substitute for medical diagnosis or professional care. It should not be implied that readers limit themselves to any one alternative medical practitioner by means of title, as many qualified and knowledgeable individuals, for a variety of reasons, may operate under different labels included under the blanket phrase of "CAM Therapy."

~Contribution by Mark Scribner

Introduction

by Joe Horn

Many people have heard the words "American health crisis epidemic" or a variation thereof thrown about in modern media. The phrase, in fact, has become so commonplace that some wouldn't even consider it breaking news. The sad reality is, however, that up to 80 percent of Americans unknowingly carry underlying medical conditions that—regardless of whether they are already experiencing symptoms—will likely eventually lead to diagnoses such as cancer, heart disease, diabetes, rheumatoid arthritis, fibromyalgia, chronic fatigue syndrome, ulcerative colitis, Crohn's disease, depression or anxiety, lupus, irritable bowel syndrome, psoriasis, eczema or other rashes, Alzheimer's disease, Lou Gehrig's disease, Parkinson's disease, hormonal or psychological imbalance, asthma, migraines, acquired food allergies, diverticulitis or diverticulosis, or many other autoimmune or inflammatory diseases.[1] Related to many of these diseases/disorders is obesity, an increasingly widespread health crisis, with two-thirds of the population in overweight standings ranging from obese to severely so.[2]

It would seem that chronic illness and obesity have hijacked the well-being of the American population.

It has been nearly twenty years since I (Joe), personally, began to see the first signs of prolonged ailment within my body. Throughout the years, I've been diagnosed by medical doctors with myriad labels: diverticulosis, diverticulitis, colonitis, irritable bowel syndrome, inflammatory bowel disease, nervous bowel disease, pleurisy, spastic colon, chronic bacterial prostatitis, nervous colon, painful bladder syndrome, epididymitis, inflamed prostate, eosinophilic esophagitis, GERD (gastroesophageal reflux disease), testosterone and infertility issues, and even genetic challenges such as MTHFR (more on this later). When my illness finally escalated in 2016 to the point that I had to have sixteen inches of my colon surgically removed, I found my hopes for a better quality of life dashed in the wake of post-surgical, ever-persisting pain that not only rivaled my pre-surgical condition, but was even worse.

The first traces of my health problem surfaced when I was a young man. At that time, I had no idea how badly I was damaging my body by working two jobs and living an otherwise sedentary lifestyle, wherein my staple food consisted of anything fast and convenient. When small, inflammatory symptoms—such as tendonitis in my wrists—appeared in my body in my early twenties, I simply wrote them off as being normal for a guitar player like myself. I remained energetic during the subsequent years, working as the activities director for a bustling camp and conference facility—a position that required me to remain in good shape physically. At six feet, three inches tall and weighing 179 pounds, I was the most fit I had ever been in my life. I was continually on the go and ate whatever I could grab between destinations. As my health began its slow decline, I attributed early symptoms to aging, fatigue, or, at times, merely "eating something that didn't settle." While, at the time, I was unaware of the medical condition brewing in my body, I *did* begin to notice two common denominators surfacing consistently: the inability to feel truly rested in the mornings, and continual digestive irregularity. Again, I attributed these symptoms to "getting older," and even when I sought help from a doctor, diet and lifestyle were never brought into question as potential causes or remedies.

I began to have chronic UTIs (urinary tract infections), which is not entirely ordinary for a man, and this brought about the first of many repetitive—and sometimes long-term—rounds of antibiotics. At this point, I was inconvenienced by these ailments, but life didn't change significantly until the night I had my first bout with E. coli—not the food-borne type, but the kind that occurred within the body as a result of a poorly functioning digestive tract. The experience was awful: I was incredibly weak, had indescribably painful chills with body aches, and experienced horrible nausea, and light hurt my eyes and head so bad that the culmination of these symptoms made it hard to move at all. I was barely able to reach the car to be driven by my wife to the hospital. Despite the doctor's willingness to link the E. coli to perhaps a small tear or ruptured polyp in my colon—for which he prescribed more antibiotics—diet and lifestyle, again, were not examined as possible culprits or solutions by the doctor.

Subsequent fertility issues that my wife and I experienced in our desire for children led to further investigation of my health and brought about a diagnosis of detrimentally low sperm count as a result of unusually high inflammation in the testicular area. Digestive issues continued to be a problem, and the tendon inflammation and ever-present fatigue remained as well. I began to encounter flare-ups of adult acne, which appeared in the form of boils all across my scalp. In addition, anxiety began to mount within me, sometimes for no apparent reason, and I would have panic attacks over events that most people would consider normal or only mildly stressful. I felt like my body ran continually on adrenalin, and, as usual, diet and lifestyle were never examined when I sought medical help.

These bouts finally escalated into events wherein I would experience sudden and debilitating chest pains, which came on so suddenly that I was certain I was having a heart attack. When I pursued treatment, the only diagnosis offered was pleurisy, which is inflammation surrounding the lungs.

Eventually, I experienced repeated events similar to those of the night I was taken to the hospital with E. coli—only in *these* instances, the symptoms were accompanied by severe abdominal pains that are difficult to describe. The verdict was that I had something called diverticulitis, a swelling and infection within polyps that form along the inside of the large intestine. The condition was explained to me as being both hereditary and common. Despite its location in my digestive tract, diet and lifestyle—*again*—were never examined by any of my doctors. Instead, I was given more antibiotics and warned that if the infection ever turned septic, it would be deadly.

In my search for remedies, I began to purchase vitamins, fiber supplements, and "healthy foods" such as celebrity-endorsed meal bars or "low-fat," salad-type groceries from big-box, corporate stores, completely unaware of their potentially harmful ingredients due to their nonorganic, commercial production. I began to eat foods that I perceived would increase my well-being, and I worked out furiously, attempting to regain fitness by "getting into better shape." The result was a sicker, more-fatigued me—who *still* suffered from all the symptoms I had previously been unable to shake. In hindsight, the only thing I did that *actually* improved my situation during that time was that I grew closer to God.

The pain and fatigue escalated to the point that it had nearly taken over my life. I searched—seemingly everywhere—for relief. The first few times my wife, Katherine, suggested natural care for my illness, I blew off the idea completely, assuming my problems were too complicated for this approach. Eventually, the gut pain landed me back in the hospital again, but this time, antibiotics brought no relief. Believing in this instance that my diverticulitis was chronic, now resistant to antibiotics, and would turn septic as the doctor had warned years previously, I pursued surgery. I believed it would be a final solution. After a desperate search for a surgeon who could see me quickly—as I was, by this time, very ill—I had an operation to remove sixteen inches of my colon.

While the surgery went smoothly, the aftermath revealed that the condition causing a great percentage of the pain had not been remedied by removing the segment of my colon. During my slow and painstaking recovery from this procedure, Katherine began to hunt for natural treatments that might change my quality of life. At first I resisted—again, believing that my problems were too convoluted to be corrected by such seemingly simple solutions. But repeatedly, more of my friends—whose input I respected greatly—joined my wife in urging me to look at natural care.

Finally, out of desperation, feeling no other paths to healing were available, I began to explore the world of natural medicine. I discovered that many ailments which, in the traditional medical realms, are labeled as "diseases" are actually addressed by natural healthcare practitioners as "imbalances" within the body that require correction. This distinction is vital! For one thing, a disease, to individuals, may feel like a permanent label they are forced to wear—one described as "hereditary," making it seem genetically unavoidable, while an "imbalance" is merely something that is currently out of place and, with the right care, could be corrected and put back in order. In addition, "diseases" are categorized by myriad symptoms that impact the body differently, and often aren't identified as being linked amongst themselves. However, many natural providers readily acknowledge that a number of disorders, when left untreated, morph into a variety of ailments that manifest throughout the physique but share the same troublesome, underlying disorder.

For example, my body was wracked with causal inflammation, which continued to show up in a variety of ways: tendonitis in my wrists; testicular irritation that caused fertility issues; swelling surrounding the lungs, producing chest pains and eventually being diagnosed as pleurisy; and, of course, the multiple chronic inflammatory diagnoses that harassed my digestive tract over the years. Furthermore, the underlying battle being fought by my adrenal system to ward off disease and restore health to my body caused an overabundance of chemical-anxiety secretion, resulting in fretfulness and panic attacks.

All of this was a result of one core, physical issue that I was never even aware of until I began my search for natural healing. That diagnosis was leaky-gut syndrome. While Western, traditional medicine provides no acknowledgment of or treatment for this condition, it is known to affect nearly 80 percent of Americans,[3] most of whom don't even realize they carry it. The ironic thing is that it doesn't always manifest in actual gut pain, therefore often goes undetected and untreated by people who later, as a result, develop some other disorder or disease. Borne largely from ingestion of processed and nonorganic foods, the condition is usually avoidable and even reversible. For many who suffer from autoimmune, neurological, or inflammatory conditions such as the extensive list at the beginning of this introduction, this underlying culprit is to blame, and a change of diet and lifestyle can reverse illness. Additionally, 80 percent of the immune system originates in the gut, so other diseases can be battled by restoring intestinal health through a change of routines and nourishment.

What I learned when I began to pursue the path of natural healing was life-changing and inspired me to recruit the assistance of Allie Anderson to write the 2018 book *Timebomb: A Genocide of Deadly Processed Foods!* My story is elaborated on throughout the book, and many aspects of the modern food crisis are explored in that work as well. If you're not familiar with that book, I encourage you to take it in. The knowledge imparted in it is vital: It is the *organic bread and butter* of information on how and why we should change our diet and heal our gut, and it provides vital information on the dangers of processed foods—which the FDA often claims are perfectly safe. Through *Timebomb*, the readers will learn about the detrimental way genetically modified and commercially farmed and produced foods, along with other elements threatening the safety of our food supply, can directly impact their personal health. But, my journey continues beyond what's included in that 2018 release, and I've discovered a wealth of additional information since then.

While gut health and the dangers of processed and genetically modified food were a great focus of my previous work, *Timebomb,* and the book is excellent for revealing the nefarious flaws in our food supply and the pharmaceutical industry, its central theme deals primarily with diet. This book, ***UNLOCKING EDEN****: Revolutionize Your Health, Maximize Your Immunity, Restore Your Vitality,* outlines additional, *essential, lifestyle changes we must make in order to achieve maximum health.* Overall well-being involves many issues beyond diet, each of which is vital to our health, and is brought to the surface in these pages.

In this work, I have partnered with Daniel Belt, CHHC (Certified Holistic Health Coach through the Institute for Integrative Nutrition, accredited by New York State University), to reveal groundbreaking information on the impact of modern society's unwitting negligence of the ways God intended for our bodies to interact with nature and how defying these principles contributes greatly to chronic illness, disease, and diminished quality of life.

Our goal is to shed light on matters that affect everybody. Those who are well and looking for preventative action will find a unique, liberating perspective from which to view your health over the course of your lifetime. If you're already ill, my ultimate prayer is that you find the way to healing through the information and suggestions we provide. However, if you don't experience what you believe to be *complete* restoration, then my supplication to God on your behalf becomes that you'll learn ways to improve the length and quality of your future.

After nearly five years of living in pursuit of natural health and being disciplined about what I put into *and* on my body, I've continued to track and achieve an entirely new quality of life. The things that Daniel and I intend to address in these pages likely won't be presented by your traditional medical physician; I know this from experience. Likewise, you probably won't hear about them from your minister at church or through your employer's wellness program. The health crisis, while urgently accelerating, has yet to be recognized by many as a life-and-death epidemic. In addition, our society has been conditioned to accept without question the answers, diagnoses, and treatment plans given by traditional medical professionals. This makes knowledge such as what we present here a rare and emergent revelation in our current culture. However, the health epidemics currently facing the masses are rampant enough that it becomes impossible to deny one truth: When large percentages of a populace seem to be sick, the culprit *must be* a common denominator. In this case, that offender is multifaceted. It includes (but isn't limited to) an under-nourishing diet, a lack of interaction with nature, an extensive exposure to toxins, and the destructively sedentary lifestyle that so many of us have become accustomed to. Unbeknownst to the average individual, devastating factors erode our ability to thrive on a daily basis. These include our lack of knowledge regarding the body's need for reliable, timed routines; overuse of our digestive tract and pancreas; broad-scale sleep deprivation; and overbooked, busy lifestyles that keep us running at full speed throughout every waking hour of the day. Many who have tackled the issue of nutritious food in their own lives believe they've taken all the measures necessary or within their power to ensure vitality. However, the principles mentioned here and throughout the rest of the book are important to thriving as well, and ignoring these matters can sabotage our best efforts at well-being. When we bring to light these detrimental, often-hidden fundamentals, we're empowered to make changes accordingly and reclaim our health, improve our quality of life, or even reverse or prevent illness.

I want to be clear that this book is about finding a pathway to the healing properties that God placed on earth for our use in pursuit of abundant life. This means that our aim is to offer guidance that will impact your lifestyle. You'll find no quick fixes in this book, and, similar to the content of *Timebomb*, the material is not based on any trending diets or exercise fads. Our desire is to point out the way to the provision of good health that has been placed within the natural realm of God's creation. These resources are often available free of charge, and they're all around. Fascinating and emergent science reveals the healing properties of even the simplest provisions God has placed in the environment. When we know where to look, we can see God's care and compassion revealed through His divine endowment. He has furnished all that we need in His creation; it's part of the birthright He has bestowed upon us!

I can't place enough emphasis on this: Regardless of your diagnosis or how ill you may be, there is hope for improvement. If you struggle with an illness or condition that you've been told is genetic or hereditary, it's possible to see, at a minimum, some reversal, because our genetics are always rewriting themselves and are constantly reacting to the environment. If you've received a medical label that involves the word "disease," it *could* be that the right diet and lifestyle changes will improve your condition or make it easier to manage—or, again, the culprit could be an imbalance that simply requires correction in order for you to see a complete reversal.

Further, I pray that this book will enrich your life and set you on a path that brings healing and hope. Just as these modifications have forever enhanced the quality of life that my family and I enjoy, I trust that you will glean knowledge that will allow you to make improvements to your own well-being and that of your family for generations to come.

~Joe Horn, fitness & nutrition specialist, COO,
Skywatch Television

chapter one

Daniel's Story

by Daniel Belt

My living room was dark, except for a ray of light that gleamed in through the window, piercing the blackness and creating a pinpoint of illumination that landed at the center of my abdomen. Surrendering to the darkness would be easy; maybe this time, I would just lie here and die. After all, I had already given up on my own life long ago. My body was still in the gloom, wracked with the severe pain and addiction to which I had become so accustomed. I no longer sought to remedy the issue with anything but that which would numb all of my senses, both physical and mental.

The music playlist shifted from an assortment of Beethoven—one of my favorites—to another of my top preferences, Bob Marley. As his song "Exodus" played, a sarcastic response crossed my mind as I heard the lyrics ask, "Are you satisfied with the life you're living?"[4]

Of course not. What kind of life is this to live, anyway?

Within just the previous few weeks, both of my maternal grandparents had passed away, and their deaths were followed by the passing of my uncle and a cousin. I had been arrested for a traffic violation that had been left unaddressed for too long, and I had spent a night in jail. When I returned from that little escapade, my girlfriend had arrived at my house to break up with me, bringing with her the surprising news that my ex-girlfriend was pregnant with my child. (Yes, you read that correctly. This was the context under which this life-altering news was delivered.) Within a week, I had lost four loved ones, experienced the humiliation of being incarcerated, continued to endure the vast physical and mental pain that had become a lifestyle, and learned that I would soon become a father.

What kind of a dad could I ever hope to be? What could I possibly have to offer to a child?

Such reflective thoughts tormented my fractured concentration as I lie there, tempted to succumb to the darkness quickly closing in on my body, my mind, my life. It was an existence I had quit fighting for, one I had given up on—thrown away, really—long ago.

I struggled, torn between a part of myself that felt my unborn child deserved my best efforts and a part that feared the fight was just too hard. I knew the one who would call me "dad" deserved a father who understood how to live an abundant life, and who would give that child a deeper and more constant connection than I had with my own father. Yet, because of the injuries and chronic pain my body had suffered as a result of chemical exposure, addiction, and extremely hard living, I wasn't sure I could ever experience what most people considered ordinary. At times, the pain had been so all-encompassing that I was unable to use my arms and legs, rendering me motionless on the floor for hours. I wondered if I ever would, or even could, get my life in order and experience normality. I knew if my child was to have the upbringing he or she needed, it was up to me to make that happen. Yet, how was I supposed to take care of someone else when I couldn't even take care of myself? Pain pulsated through my body, tormenting me. Feelings of worthlessness tortured my mind, daring me to just give up.

How I do move forward from here?

As I languished in this valley of decision between fighting and relinquishing the battle for my life, the song on the player changed, and another Marley tune began to play. This song was "Get Up, Stand Up." It was as though I was hearing the words for the first time, as though God Himself were answering my question. I knew that He was telling me to get up and fight. My answer came clearly in that moment. I looked toward the pinprick of light glowing on my abdomen and heard the words: "So now you see the light… Stand up for your rights."[5] God was speaking to me, ordering me to take action. Now. I could feel Him working in my being. A change was taking place in my spirit, even though the physical pain remained. Slowly, and despite physical agony, I began to follow instructions. I climbed to my feet. Finally, after years of tremendous and debilitating pain that had left me incapacitated physically and mentally, I was ready to believe in a better existence. God had spoken to me, and He saw value in me. He would help me. For the first time, I fully surrendered the pain to God. In faith, I stood up, ready to work for the life I had previously been willing to throw away.

As this change took place, a new charge permeated my mind. God showed me a revelation that rippled throughout my core being, and my attention was recalled to every wounded warrior I had met at the Veterans Affairs (VA) hospitals as a soldier recovering from injuries I had sustained during my military training. I thought of every person whose path I had crossed—and who, like me, struggled with chronic pain. But most of all, I remembered each individual who had shared my own all-too-familiar lack of hope. Righteous indignation on behalf of those tormented souls began to burn within me, inciting in my being a new mission, a fresh sense of purpose. As I surrendered to that drive, my eyes opened to the spiritual warfare taking place around me. The pinpoint of light maintained its steady placement within the room as the darkness at the corners of the area grew black. Demonic entities clamoring for a grip on my well-being—on my very soul—began grasping in my direction, frantically reaching to maintain control over my destiny.

But it was too late! God had already given me a new direction, imbued me with new determination, and imparted a new assignment on my previously despondent existence. I thought of the multitudes suffering with chronic pain and illness—those for whom it seemed there was no hope of a better life—and in an instant, I was compelled to help them.

The words God spoke to me echoed through my mind as though they had been audible: "You won't be defeated by the pain. Stand up. There's work to do."

I was born in the 1970s. My mom was an unwed teenager who had the courage to give birth to me—an unexpected challenge during her youth. She did her best, and throughout her multiple marriages, there were periods when I lived with my maternal and paternal grandparents, as well as a short time with my dad. I watched Mom struggle in nearly every way: financially, socially, relationally, and even within the church, where her lifestyle suffered intense scrutiny by legalistic attendees. My mindset began to orient itself at a very young age toward hatred for hypocrisy, cruelty, and injustice—all the attitudes and behaviors I had watched victimize my mother. In fact, I saw her suffer so greatly at the hands of those who claimed Christianity that, when I was eight—after reading about Buddhism's themes of self-accountability and finding that logic attractive—I privately converted to that worldview for a time. I was attracted to the notion that there were people who not only would recognize a higher power, but who would also self-manage accountability and behaviors in a way that facilitated a search for light, love, and harmony.

As a kid, I struggled with self-esteem, but compensated with a nonchalant, egotistical demeanor. I shored up areas I felt I was lacking in with knowledge, which I then used to feed my pride to make up for deficiencies. I saw myself as an agent for justice by beating up bullies and befriending the underdogs. I was athletic, excelled at sports, and was always physically active. I spent lunch break and recesses at school running or otherwise engaging in physical exertion, as I did on afternoons, evenings, and weekends. My childhood spare time nearly always involved playing outside.

My maternal grandparents were very kind and good to me, although their fire-and-brimstone approach to religion caused me to shy away at times. In response, I found myself averting my thoughts from eternity— or even my own earthly future, for that matter—to adopt a focus on the here and now over everything else. As I grew older with that attitude, my active, always-on-the-go lifestyle morphed into running around on the streets as a teenager—drinking, using recreational drugs, and partying as though there were no tomorrow.

For most of my childhood, as I said, I drifted between the homes of my mother and maternal grandparents, with occasional time spent with my dad. He was a kind man with a heart of gold, but he never could seem to commit to anything, let alone apply himself to full-time fatherhood. This had been tough while I was little, but as I grew older, we were able to engage in activities such as hunting, camping, and fishing. Dad was always quite the outdoorsman, capable of sustaining himself on what nature provided. As a matter of fact, one day he said he was tired of the noise of the city; he moved out to the country and never looked back. From that day on, for the rest of his life, he lived off the land.

At seventeen, I was ready to turn over a new leaf. I had watched my mother struggle financially, and I was tired of poverty. I wanted more than anything to be educated, to have the power to create good opportunities for myself. I dreamed of being articulate, of traveling the world, and of forging paths of fortune that would distance me from the underprivileged life I had grown ashamed of. Every man in my dad's family up to this point had served in the US Army, and I wanted to make him proud of me—a desire I later learned was a typical response for a child with a distant-father relationship. I was only a high school junior, but already lived on my own, working nights at Taco Bell. I enrolled for the "split option," which enabled me to join the National Guard the summer after my junior year to complete basic training, then return home to attend my senior year of high school with the plan to continue military service after graduation. While this fed my need to be empowered and propel my own life's direction, it created a wedge between myself and my peers, because it felt similar to revisiting childhood after stepping outside of it. I felt like a fish out of water, waiting to get back to my newer, bigger, better pond.

After I graduated, I went into the Army, where I had several assignments. The one I eventually settled into was that of an Apache helicopter crew chief in Kentucky with the 101st Airborne. I was also part of the air assault division, which required that I master repelling out of helicopters, conquer obstacle courses, and accomplish other feats of strength that are hard on the body. The Army is required to train its personnel to do massive amounts of physical work on little sleep while sustaining on MRE ("meal, ready-to-eat"; meal replacement/protein) bars, and sometimes enduring feats of chemical exposure. While the Army does attempt to take all precautions possible where safety and exposure are concerned, it simply isn't possible to train soldiers without imposing some degree of risk.

By this time, my previously wild lifestyle had followed me into the service. I was heavily involved in drinking and drugs, yet functioned like a well-oiled machine during the day, fulfilling all responsibilities required of me while partying late into—or through—the night. I lived as though I had a death wish. I ate voraciously, paying no attention to calories or any other intake marker, and drank as many eight to ten soft drinks per day. I worked all day, then at night used any combination of ecstasy, LSD, and/or cocaine while heavily drinking a variety of hard liquors. Then I followed up the inundation of chemical inebriates with such activities as nightclubbing, running around on the streets, or even repelling—all while I was under the influence. One stunt my buddies and I engaged in was what we called "Aussie-style repelling": We would jump from the top of a repel point, head-first, to see who could get the closest to the ground before abruptly stopping the downward motion. There were many times I hurt myself brutally—breaking several bones, including my ribs, clavicle, arms, and even both hands and ankles. The injuries caused horrific pain, but fueled by my lust for adrenalin, I continued the escapades. There were several mornings after such nights that I returned to work never having slept at all. Having years before relinquished my short-termed stint in Buddhism, I held no religious views at this time. The fruitlessness of my search created a hostility that slowly turned inward, causing me to wish for my own destruction.

One day, I was participating in a mock-wartime drill where troops are told to pack their provisions and round up as though headed for combat, then they're assigned a territory to occupy and defend. We arrived at the delegated zone and the exercise began. I was in a prone position on the ground (as a soldier on his or her belly, either preparing to crawl or with a gun positioned for fire) when a gas canister landed about three feet in front of me. I saw a stream of smoke coming out of it, but had no time to respond before it jettisoned a substance straight into my face, hitting me at eye level. I had on no mask—no protection whatsoever. My memory of what happened next is vague. Frankly, it's traumatic to try to remember. I do recall that fluid was coming from my nostrils, mouth, and eyes. The pain was indescribable. Before I blacked out completely, I remember trying to run. When I returned to consciousness, I was lying on a cot in the on-location clinic. My memory fades in and out, but I know I was soon moved to the base office for further examination. For days during this period, my vision was foggy and the events seemed to defy chronology. The quality of my recollection of the remainder of my days in the service leaves intermittent, gaping holes in my mind's storyline.

The incident was never officially recognized. When I inquired about the type of gas or chemical I had been exposed to, my query was simply dismissed—no answers. However, I soon began to notice a physical change after that incident. While areas of my body that had previously been wounded began to hurt more than they had in the past, new capacities for aching emerged where there had never even been an injury. I began to develop nerve pain, which could be slow at the onset or very sudden. The discomfort was always debilitating and seemed to respond to no method of relief. Additionally, my body appeared to be weakened; activities that shouldn't have hurt me resulted in injuries that incapacitated me. This wasn't only physically agonizing, but was also demoralizing for a young man who, until now, had been strong and able-bodied—almost challenging fate to send him a conquest he could not tackle. As VA clinics and hospitals continued to maintain that I hadn't suffered chemical exposure, it soon became obvious that this was beside the point. Regardless of the cause, they still had no idea how to treat my pain. Speculative diagnoses involved terms such as ankylosing spondylosis, MLPB (mechanical lower back pain), and fibromyalgia. Some physicians even offered such seemingly unrelated theories as high cholesterol and blood pressure, insomnia, and chronic fatigue syndrome. The more unrelated the diagnosis seemed, the more obvious it became that the medical team was grasping at straws to pinpoint the enigmatic nature of the nerve-related pain.

During this time, my previous compulsion to party, drink heavily, and consume any mixed cocktail of street drugs and prescription meds began to take on a more desperate undertone. What had previously been recreational now derived from my need to manage the uncontrollable pain. Soon, in addition to my other ailments, I was suffering from a prescription pain medication addiction. Unfortunately, the agony was only vaguely shrouded by the combination of heavy medications and alcohol. It was a hopeless place to be. I was dealing with chronic pain, coupled with the increasing inability to mask the anguish, alongside having doctor after doctor unable to tell me what was happening to my body. Nobody was even able to narrow the diagnosis down to a potential culprit. Caution and thinking preventatively didn't help the situation, either; I would continue to hurt terribly where there was no injury.

I became angry. I blamed doctors for their inability to diagnose or treat me. Fractures in my self-esteem that I had previously subsidized with feats of bravado or physical achievement were now exposed and sensitive, reminding me of the man I used to be. I had always been strong and resourceful. Worst of all, my symptoms seemed to come and go in a pendulum-type fashion: One day, week, or month, I'd feel great, only to have the awful pain return and incapacitate me again. Such periods of relief only served as teasers of the life I was now being robbed of. Additionally, these spurts made my social dynamic awkward with peers. Many of the people I worked with couldn't understand why, on a particular day, I would be incapable of something I had done easily only a week before. It was infuriating and flabbergasting. My body had never failed me like this. As coping became tougher, I was placed on antidepressants in addition to pain meds.

During this time, my lowest emotional moments seemed equal to the depths of the sea, only to be followed by the highs that were brought on when physical pain was relieved, giving me a glimpse into the life I could be living. However, these heights were always followed by the pain—thus, the depths—of this "pain-pendulum" having swung the other direction yet again. My self-hate and guilt hit an all-time high, fueled by the recollection of my younger days when I had held such noble values as justice, accountability, and authenticity. I detested who I had become. Now, there were nights that I stretched out on my floor unable to move and in so much pain I couldn't even read. I felt worthless, lonely, even isolated, and my self-loathing convinced me I deserved to feel this way. Any relationship I became involved in, I quickly sabotaged. Overwhelmed with my inability to measure up to standards I had set for myself earlier in life, I succumbed to my rage and gave up. I developed a "why even try?" attitude, which I employed in self-destructive activities such as using more drugs, drinking more alcohol, and indulging in a new deviant streak that allowed me to lie, cheat, commit indiscretions, and behave against my previously held moral codes. The physical pain was so intense that I just didn't care anymore.

Throughout this entire time, doctors continued to prescribe medications to mask my symptoms, but since they were unable to target the issue causing the agony, they offered no real solutions. They never examined my diet, exercise, or lifestyle to find remedies. As the pain increased and eventually became unbearable, my hope of a normal life continued to diminish until the possibility seemed nonexistent. Finally, I decided to further drown the mental, emotional, and physical anguish with drugs and alcohol, knowing it was likely only a matter of time before they finished me off completely. I was aware that the direction I was heading would eventually become fatal, but I had no more will to fight. My desire to live was gone, and instead, I settled for the concept of numbing the aching on my way out of this world.

Living in this manner, it wasn't long before, one night, under the influence of many chemical substances, I sat reflecting about the direction my life had taken. I was tired, jaded, and disenchanted with my existence—far removed from the idealistic young man who had made it his mission to beat up bullies and befriend the underdogs. This had been a particularly rough day; a dear friend had attempted suicide, and my intervention had stopped it. My heart was broken, I felt confused and directionless, and, as usual, I was wracked with pain.

———

As I sat there, I had a vision: Everything went dark. I saw myself walking in the blackness. There appeared to be no ground before me, but each time I placed a foot forward in a stepping motion, a glowing green stone would rise from the murky abyss below and position itself beneath my foot. Each time I would place my weight on the boulder, a memory from my life would play out before me like a movie. Sins I had committed played out in gruesome detail. Every dirty or underhanded deed I had ever been a part of—each violent, cheating, solicitous thing I had ever done—I now relived in a vivid accounting. Even events I had completely forgotten were now revealed in stark detail. Each step forward into the blackness brought a new, illuminated stone to suspend itself before my foot just in time to catch me, and with it came a new and tormenting memory of my deeds.

Yet, with each step I took, a rock was left behind me as I continued walking forward, placing one foot in front of the other. Every time I pulled my foot from one stone to proceed to the next, the one behind me would shatter into a million pieces and disappear, and a light would flash on my forehead, bringing with it a memory of something good about my life. Some of these revelations were memories of times I had shown compassion or committed acts of love for other people, while others were affirmations of positive attributes that I held. With every boulder that disintegrated behind me, I was reminded that I was loved, that there was virtue in me, and that God saw me as someone who was worth saving. Until this moment, I had always seen God as the One reflected in the harsh judgment of my mother's fellow churchgoers. I had perceived myself as unworthy of love or salvation, as though my shortcomings needed continual compensation or negotiation.

However, that wasn't how God saw me at all.

In this moment, God was sending me this vital message: You have made mistakes, but they don't define you. I see the good in you, and I love you. The past, like these stones, has fallen away and lies behind you—but—you must step forward into your calling in order to live out the good things I have for you.

———

Allow me to be clear, because I can't emphasize this enough: In that single moment, my understanding of who Jesus is and how He wanted to work in my life was embryonic. The profoundness of the message downloaded into me—in that isolated instant—literally took years to unpack. In fact, it is still, even now, being revealed to me in new ways all the time. Jesus spoke to me both on a level I was able to grasp at that time, and also in volumes that would unfold over subsequent years as my relationship with Him grew. While I had previously been philosophically aware of Jesus in a scholarly way, the Person He wanted to be in my own life opened my ability to see Him in a new light. Until then, my perception of Jesus had been skewed and underdeveloped. But that moment was the beginning of Him correcting decades of my misperceptions of Him, launching a series of revelations that continue even until this day.

As I reemerged into reality, I wasn't yet sure what to do with that information. I remembered the stories of salvation I had heard as a child, and I knew without doubt that God had spoken to me. However, it was still difficult to wrap my brain around the concept that God had reassured me of the good He saw in me. And, despite the fact that the vision had clearly communicated that I was supposed to move forward, I wasn't yet certain of how to go about it. While it was clear that God wanted me to change my life, I was still assessing where to even begin. I kept an open mind as I proceeded through the next few days, knowing that change was both necessary and imminent. I watched for an opportunity to begin the process.

The subsequent days brought the culmination of events I mentioned at the beginning of the chapter: That traffic violation I had not addressed finally caught up with me, necessitating a night in jail. As I mourned the death of several loved ones, I lost a girlfriend and learned I was going to be a father. By now, it had only been a few days since the vision involving the stones, and I lie on my floor contemplating how to go about the revolution I knew God was ordering in my life. The change had been initiated, but it wasn't until that little pinprick of light settled over my abdomen as God spoke to me that I truly began to believe. As I recalled all the hurting individuals with whom I had made contact over the course of my own search for healing, Bob Marley's words, "Get up, stand up,"[6] resonated in my ears. God's message pounded through my being: "You won't be defeated by the pain. Stand up. There's work to do." Despite the fact that Marley was a secular artist, God used his music to set my life on a fresh course. My new mission solidified in my spirit, and I found a fresh strength for the pursuit of healing—not only for myself, but for others who needed help as well. *In that single moment, God inscribed a calling upon my heart.*

While it took all my strength to stand due to the physical torment involved, I did so, determined to follow the new direction God was placing on my life. I knew He was telling me to clean my house and restore my previously held, higher standards, to get rid of everything that was brought into my setting without intention. Items, habits, and even relationships that had simply meandered into my existence because of my complacent standards were removed as I struggled to bring my new charge into focus. I quit every bad habit cold-turkey: drugs, alcohol, prescription medications, etc.

I would love to say that God miraculously healed all my pain, but that is not the case. Instead, what He did was begin to illuminate Scripture and impart knowledge to me while bolstering my strength in correlation with each day's struggles. He gave me conviction that reminded me daily—in no uncertain terms—that I needed to understand His laws and live His way. This, to me, went farther than following His biblical commandments (which we are called to do), and extended into understanding His creation and how our bodies align within it. I knew I had to find a natural way to heal my body rather than keep turning to medications that were addictive and only disguised my symptoms. It became vital to understand the provision that God had included in the earth He created and placed us within, and how the harmony between the two creates a balance of health that is our birthright as His creation.

It was a tough chapter. I contended with raw, unmasked physical pain while stepping out in the faith it took to adopt this new lifestyle. As God incrementally bestowed knowledge, I made progress against the physical pain. My commitment to follow Him and live according to His will throughout all phases of my search for healing continually strengthened. Looking back, I see that even when I didn't yet understand the science revealing why something was in my best interest, God's prompting still led me in the right direction because I was seeking Him. Slowly, He reminded me of the visits I had spent with my dad and how he had taught me to live off the land. I remembered the peace, joy, and provision my dad had found in the rural, self-sustained setting. He had taught me to hunt and fish, and how to clean, catch, and cook my own food. On a few occasions, we camped for weeks at a time, only eating what nature provided. Despite the distant quality of my relationship with my father throughout my childhood years, I realized that he had given me a priceless gift in the lessons I learned during those visits. It shows that God is one of grace and mercy. Even when we are without the tools required to help ourselves, He sets His plan for us into place.

Soon, I began to work at a store specializing in organic foods and supplements in an effort to learn by proximity: If I had a job in a setting where people knew about natural health, surely I would eventually be knowledgeable, too. However, I soon realized that I was surrounded by people who had just as many questions as I had, and many were fighting terrible illnesses. Their search for relief was desperate. I was astounded to realize that the health epidemic in our society had hit crisis levels. Further, there were people asking me for help who, in my opinion, shouldn't have been as sick as they were; many were young and should have appeared strong and healthy. I quickly realized that there is no pattern—age, income bracket, or predictable "candidates"—for the manifestation of an ailment. It's hard to reconcile this, since America has more medical interventions available than many other countries. You'd think that we'd be the healthiest population in the world, with only a few exceptions. But, I soon found the opposite to be the case, and my desire to help people only grew. My mission to find relief was rekindled, and the boy inside me who wanted to stand up for the underdog sought answers—not only for myself, but for these folks as well. Many reported multiple, or even conflicting, diagnoses that had become the outcome of a fruitless search for answers within the medical world. Interestingly, a number of these people talked to me in ways they apparently didn't use when talking to their doctors. They were candid, strategic, even desperate when we discussed their medical issues. Each story I heard sparked a new search for solutions in the natural healing world.

The more I hunted for and prayed for remedies, the more I discovered that while there seemed to be limitless manifestations of illness, the triggers of sickness were less varied. In fact, there seemed to be a somewhat predictable pattern related to many disorders and diseases. Things such as diet, lifestyle, even quality of life surfaced as elements that could be considered preventative. I realized that simple things our culture gives no thought to, such as depriving ourselves of interaction with nature, can create chemical imbalances within our systems that make essential functions like metabolism or detox processes nearly impossible. We've also adopted many practices that impede the body's ability to care for itself, such as the way we stunt our immune system's ability to develop and operate at full capacity by the large-scale use of products such as pesticides and antibiotics.

Throughout this time, the Lord continued to reveal simple principles for which I would only later find the supporting science. For example, I knew my pain would ease if I went back to the kinds of streams where my dad and I fished together. I didn't know *how* it would work; I only knew that it would. Later, I learned that exposing the body to cold, moving water triggers a response called mitochondrial biogenesis, which initiates the rejuvenation and repopulation of healthy cells (more on this in an upcoming chapter). By making such discoveries and learning about the science that supports them, I began to realize that the lifestyle of many Americans is self-destructive and predisposes us to become ill. Simultaneously, we remain unaware of the healing properties available in creation, which has been given to us for our use and to bless us with health (Genesis 1:26–30). This was given to us freely by the One who made it and owns it, and its access and use is our birthright as part of God's creation. Best of all, many of the things that have the power to heal us are free and readily available, once we know where to look.

The Bible speaks of many natural elements that most people interpret as metaphorical, but that I believe are literal as well. For example, the first gift mankind was given was the breath of life, breathed into Adam by God Himself, as he was created (Genesis 2:7). When we understand the power of clean air, this gains significance. Similarly, "light" is frequently referred to in Scripture as a positive, healing, or even saving entity (Matthew 4:16, 5:16; John 8:12; James 1:17). Such passages seem to have a literal in addition to a spiritual element, considering the science supporting the vast health benefits of sunlight. I've already mentioned that fresh, flowing water can help detox and heal the body, so it shouldn't surprise us that God Himself refers "pure water" (Hebrews 10:22), and "living water" (Zechariah 14:8). The list of comparisons goes on and on, but we can also see that God likens things that are unhealthy to the most dry and desolate places found on earth (Psalm 68:6; Jeremiah 17:6; Ezekiel 19:13). Perhaps the most convincing argument regarding God's view of our intentional placement within natural creation can be found in Genesis 1, which states that Adam and Eve were placed in a garden as the manifestation of God's will for mankind's existence.

The earth is filled with resources to help us acquire and maintain healthy lives; the key is awareness of the gifts available. Hosea 4:6 warns that we will perish "for lack of knowledge." God has given us instructions for how to navigate the search for spiritual truths; we can follow the same guidelines in our search for health and healing:

> According as his divine power hath given unto us all things that pertain unto life and godliness, through the knowledge of him that hath called us to glory and virtue: Whereby are given unto us exceeding great and precious promises: that by these ye might

be partakers of the divine nature, having escaped the corruption that is in the world through lust. And beside this, giving all diligence, add to your faith virtue; and to virtue knowledge; And to knowledge temperance; and to temperance patience; and to patience godliness; And to godliness brotherly kindness; and to brotherly kindness charity. (2 Peter 1:3–7)

This passage explains that we've been given great power pertaining to life and godliness through the wisdom God imparts. Precious promises are available to those who will transcend earthly lusts and be diligent in faith and virtue. We're told to add knowledge to this, followed by temperance (self-control), patience, godliness, brotherly kindness, and finally, charity (love).

This is a list of vital instructions. It begins with faith and the willingness to seek what is good. When we've found those two resources, we're to begin our pursuit of information, an endeavor that will feed the subsequent characteristics listed, up to and including love. This is an order from our Creator that directs our standard of living. It's about pursuing health and quality of life, helping each other, chasing holistic peace, and living abundantly.

My journey hasn't been an easy road—and even today, I'm not completely pain-free. The difference is that I no longer mask the aching; instead, I use my physical challenges as fuel for the unending pursuit of healing. When we have completely broken free of something, we often move on and forget the victory we've been given. Instead, that which remains as a reminder becomes the source of unwavering determination to continue the battle. My discomfort has become manageable, and the discipline I must live with in order to maintain it serves the same resolve as the one that feeds the drive toward my mission and my calling.

Few individuals read medically themed, nonfiction works out of mere curiosity or for entertainment. Nearly everyone who picks up a book like this has is a personal motivation to learn about the subject. Perhaps you, the reader, have been told that you or a loved one has a chronic or auto-immune illness such as Alzheimer's, Parkinson's, Crohn's, diabetes, multiple sclerosis, chronic fatigue syndrome, digestive disorders, or an inflammatory illness such as arthritis. Or, maybe you're seeking insight regarding depression or anxiety. While traditional medicine offers treatments for many symptoms of these ailments, it often provides little hope of a cure—let alone the inspiration to believe it's possible to enjoy a high quality of life under such circumstances. Yet, God has designed prevention and/or relief for many of these issues through the providential beauty of His creation. And, as stated previously, these remedies are often found, free of charge, in the places we have access to by simply pursuing the natural world surrounding us each day.

The words of Jesus Himself are a testament to the fact that He wants to give us a peaceful and restful existence. When we have surrendered all to our Creator, He wants our lives to be free of heartache and lived in the harmonious rest of a worry-free life:

Come unto me, all ye that labour and are heavy laden, and I will give you rest. Take my yoke upon you, and learn of me; for I am meek and lowly in heart: and ye shall find rest unto your souls. For my yoke is easy, and my burden is light. (Matthew 11:28–30)

Unfortunately, many who begin the journey toward natural care quickly immerse themselves in strenuous exercise routines, excessive supplement intake, or binge purchases of products labeled "health foods" without understanding what makes them so. While measures like these, at times, can enhance well-being or recovery from physical ailments, they cannot be the sole solutions to illness. The key is found in adopting a lifestyle that addresses the entire body and reconnects the physical and emotional condition to that of creation.

Additionally, I'd like to echo Joe's words to make it clear that you won't find any quick fixes in the upcoming pages. This book offers no trendy, fad diets, and there are no get-skinny-quick schemes within these pages. Instead, Joe and I will provide information about the free and readily available pathways toward natural healing that exist around us at every turn. To repeat: God intends for us to live in abundance and walk in healing, and He has provided the means for health in the earth that He created for us. It is my hope that as you read this book, you will rediscover the love bestowed upon you by your Maker through the meticulous care that He has surrounded you with.

The value of how we feel physically and mentally are commonly traded for what we perceive as our immediate needs, and this is often done to our own demise (this is why industries such as predatory lending and fast food thrive). Joe and I plan to address this by providing basic knowledge and wisdom that we have walked away from—the gifts that are humanity's birthright.

We care deeply about your daily life. The premise of our platform is to strengthen your knowledge of the tools available to empower you with control over your life. One of the greatest obstacles to living a strong and vital life is a lack of clarity regarding how to pursue health. Often, we suffer because we simply can't see what we need to make our lives better. To this end, we'll simplify and distill the basic aspects of what it means to live well. In my view, an essential ingredient of quality of life then becomes *choice*. It gives us conviction to truly understand our decisions, because we either make them intentionally or as a byproduct of complacency or habit. Since so many people have limited knowledge of how their own bodies and the natural world work, the absence of intentional living often has a profoundly negative effect on their health. The lifestyle we propose takes time and commitment, but can provide lasting well-being. Furthermore, emerging science reinforces everything we're presenting.

If you or a loved one are fighting illness, I implore you to read these pages with an open mind and a prayerful heart. Your story is still being written, and whatever obstacle, disorder, or disease you've been told is encrypted in your genetic code, allow me to encourage you: This is not your final prognosis. You have the ability to change the quality of your life and possibly even lengthen it. As you take in the information provided in this book, please remember that regardless of what health challenges you or those dear to you may be facing, the story isn't finished. The fact that you're reading this book is testament to your willingness to make efforts toward victory.

Your story is still being written.

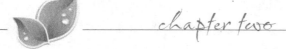

chapter two

Conditioned Culture

"Doctor Knows Best"

When we begin to search for ways to foster well-being through natural approaches, one of the first challenges we face is having family, peers, or others offer negative opinions about this journey. For many, leaning on natural elements seems too simple to hold the keys to solving complex medical concerns. However, we wish to challenge this thinking: Why shouldn't our bodies benefit most from a gentle, natural approach? Why should harsh pharmaceuticals and chemicals (which often have detrimental side effects) *always* be our first resort? Further, why is the success of natural remedies never touted in the news or on social media? This indicates that our society has migrated toward buying quick fixes for many ailments and unquestioningly submitting to the authority of those prescribing these solutions, rather than investing in their overall well-being across the span of their lifetimes—even when they aren't experiencing discomfort or illness.

For example, founder of CHT Wellness' signature program, Wholistic Blueprint, Cynthia Thurlow, recognizes that many would rather remedy their obesity problems with a pill than with a fitness-oriented approach. "It makes me want to cry," she says, "when my female patients would prefer I write them a prescription than work on changing their diet, [engage in] more exercise, [or take on] other lifestyle changes."[7] Yet, shortcuts such as pharmaceuticals are taken every day, with side effects disregarded and overall wellness shoved to a back burner—and too many follow without question, at the expense of their health, the professionals who facilitate these practices.

Unfortunately, many within our modern society are conditioned to subject themselves to authority. This becomes cyclical, in that the more we outsource the care of our own health, the more we must lean on those whom we perceive to be experts on our well-being. The image portrayed to a consumer or patient, however, doesn't always carry the promised merit. For example, actors or models *hired* to pose in lab coats are often the ones we place our trust in as we buy products labeled with claims of bettering our well-being. As a result, we embrace foods, supplements, and even pharmaceuticals based on our impression (and thus, trust) of such characters who, in *real life*, may have no credibility, training, or authority to make such recommendations (more on this in a bit).

When it comes to those who *have* had medical training, such as healthcare workers, doctors, and surgeons, we often obey them without question simply because we perceive them to be "in the know." Consider the number of times you may have heard an acquaintance speak of taking a medication that either manifested a dangerous side effect or counteracted another one he or she was taking. The results of these side effects and interactions can range from inconvenient to potentially fatal. Even when a doctor has thoroughly researched and vetted a medication, the product may have hidden secondary effects that haven't yet been discovered or reported.

In any such instance, the reason for taking the drug always seems to be the same: "The doctor told me to."

Dangerously Conditioned

Our society is so dangerously inclined to blindly follow the orders of attending physicians that there's a record of many instances when patients or even subordinate healthcare professionals go against their own instinct or training to follow the superiors' orders.

It is unfortunate that, as we go about our daily lives giving little or no thought to the preventative care of our bodies, we elevate medical professionals so highly: We expect them to solve complex medical issues that are often the product of *our own* self-neglect. We perceive them to be capable of healing us should the need arise; in this way, we avoid having to take responsibility for our own health. We imagine physicians as some type of "safety net," with unlimited resources and vast knowledge that will surely bail us out should we find ourselves ill. Not only is this false thinking, but it puts us in the unfortunate position of placing godlike expectations upon mere human beings. In response, we surrender authority to them.

An extreme example of this submission-to-authority dynamic can be found in a highly controversial experiment conducted by Stanley Milgram at Yale University in the early 1960s (we'll elaborate on the relevance between this experiment and our current topic in the upcoming pages). In this study, volunteers were recruited to participate in what they were told was a learning experiment. In truth, the study focused on individuals' propensity to obey authority figures and the researchers' desire to see just how far a participant would go to remain compliant. (The ethics of this study were subsequently called into question, for good reason, but it nonetheless illustrates a willingness to obey authority figures even if it goes against one's inclination.)

The experiment worked like this:

Volunteers were assigned the role of "teachers," and believed the "students" were participants in the study as well. The *represented* premise for this research (not the *real* one) was to test memory retention when it's reinforced by punishment. This was (supposedly) assured by an electric shock applied when volunteers asked to recall information gave incorrect answers. However, these "students" were actors pretending to convulse in pain when they were "shocked" for giving a wrong answer. The unsuspecting "teachers" were instructed to relay two words to their counterparts, who supposedly would attempt to remember the words in order to avoid the punishment. When the time came for recall, if the "students" didn't remember the elements of the memory test, the "teachers" were to administer the penalty, a consequence technique said to increase learning, thus (supposedly) making this step a vital part of the process.

This discipline was administered by requiring participants to press a series of buttons they were told delivered voltage. The severity of surges was labeled on the mechanism in these increments: "Slight Shock," "Very Strong Shock," "Danger: Severe Shock," and even "XXX."[8] As the number of incorrect answers given by the "students" (recall that the volunteers were unaware that they were dealing with actors) increased, the volunteers were instructed to administer shocks in mounting levels of intensity. As the power of the shocks escalated, those receiving the punishment would complain that the pain was becoming more intense. Eventually, the actors would be screaming, even stating the desire for the experiment to end and saying that they no longer wanted to participate. At times, some would refuse to answer the questions, supposedly afraid they would give the wrong response and be shocked again. However, the conductors (individuals in charge) instructed volunteers to treat non-responses as wrong answers; this caused volunteers to have to administer severe shocks to people who did not respond.

This experiment may seem cruel and manipulative. Certainly, many of Milgram's critics thought so, and his practices weren't condoned during subsequent scrutiny. To be truthful, his career never was the same when his methods were revealed. But we can still gain valuable knowledge from the research (although we are saddened by the trauma it surely caused his volunteers). Usually, those asked to predict what they would do in such a situation would assert their refusal to initiate or continue administering shocks as the intensity escalated, yet surprisingly, *two-thirds* of Milgram's participants remained obedient *all the way through the experiment*: Two out of three continued to send electrical surges past the time when the "student" asked for the procedure to stop, beyond the point of becoming completely unresponsive and even to the place that he or she was directed to administer the maximum voltage, which was said to equal *450 volts*.[9]

Milgram noted visual signs of inner conflict among participants, such as "sweating, trembling, stuttering, biting their lips, and so on," but despite this, they still yielded authority to those they perceived to be the "experts" or "in charge."[10] The experimenter found similar results when conducting the same study but with one variation: At the beginning of the procedure, the individual receiving the voltage mentioned having a heart condition. Even with this, the percentage of people who followed the order to deal out shocks was 62.5 percent.[11] Also interesting is that when the experimenter left the room and instead gave orders over a telephone, the obedience rate dropped by 20.5 percent.[12] This indicates that the physical presence of the authoritative figure while giving orders has an impact on the subordinate's compliance.

To further identify factors that may have contributed to obedience, Milgram relocated to a shabby office and conducted the experiments again there to see if the willingness to follow orders had anything to do with the participants' esteem for Yale University. The obedience rate reduced to 47.5 percent.[13] This means that in addition to proximity of the actual authority figure, the participants' opinion of the professional setting lent credibility to the commands.

Through this effort, Milgram was trying to explain why in circumstances such as the Holocaust or the My Lai Massacre in Vietnam, when soldiers killed hundreds of civilians, those following orders would be compelled to obey beyond what their morality would ordinarily allow. As stated earlier, Milgram's methods were criticized by his comrades, who said that the experiment had no "external validity,— [in other words, the results could not be] generalized to other situations and other people" as it pertained to the willingness to inflict pain on another human being, merely to follow orders.[14]

However, what this experiment *did* show is brought to light by another critic of Milgram: "Participants in an experiment are concerned with being good subjects and acting in a manner that they perceive is expected of them."[15] They were told that their "students" would receive no permanent physical damage by trusted influences such as the experimenter, who, during some of the sessions, appeared as a representative of the esteemed Yale University.

Disclaimer

Certainly, the controversial nature of this experiment should be considered before assuming that what we can learn from it can be flawlessly leaned upon. We're not asserting that the methodology was without fault. Yet, there are elements worth correlating to our psyche as patients. For one thing, participants in this process maintained between a 47.5 to 62.5 obedience rate, despite the fact that they *believed themselves to be* creating discomfort on their "student." (Milgram obtained other percentages of compliance/disobedience by subsequently varying the procedure significantly from the one that has been discussed here.) The fact that individuals were willing to follow such instructions likely stemmed from three primary elements:

1. They didn't believe they were inflicting permanent, physical damage to the "learner."
2. A figure of authority told them their actions were necessary for the "memory study," and thus contributed to the general betterment of society via knowledge gleaned.

3. The participants' compliance was a reflection of their esteem of the facility or qualifications of the individuals hosting the procedure.

At this point you may be wondering how a psychological test nearly six decades old and conducted by a man with questionable methods could *possibly* be relevant in today's world. As we've admitted, there are flaws in the concept of leaning *completely* on this experiment to make our argument. Yet, this study *does* demonstrate some timeless truths:

1) People often obey instructions—even those that go against their own instincts—when someone in authority tells them they are necessary or good.
2) The credibility of the *facility* represented adds motivation to the willingness to submit to authority.
3) People frequently perceive a beneficial outcome to be worth the endurance of pain.

When we apply these truths to current attitudes toward healthcare, we can easily see that a large percentage of the populace readily farms out the responsibility for their healthcare to people who seem professional, appear knowledgeable, and work in facilities we have confidence in. Additionally, we tend to trust specialists who use the latest equipment, who have access to the largest and most up-to-date inventory of pharmaceuticals, and who seem to speak in language that demonstrates a solid working knowledge of the subject matter.

Often, those seeking medical care are overwhelmed by their symptoms and assume that professionals know more about their body than they do. Regardless of how society came to be this way, the vast majority of Americans completely count on our doctors to make our healthcare decisions. As surprising as it may seem, the mentality that Milgram's study unearthed still thrives in the undercurrent of psychology as it pertains to medical care.

It is an unfortunate fact that we live in a "doctor knows best" setting, where a large percentage of those living in our communities are content to farm out healthcare decisions to those they perceive to have both unlimited knowledge and the power to save them. Consider the trend of leaving specialized pursuits up to the "experts." This is how we purchase our food, obtain home and car repairs, file our taxes, secure legal direction—it's how we do *everything*. It would seem that the details of taking proactive care of our health has become an inconvenience we hardly afford the time for. In other words, we delegate the maintenance or repair of everything—including our own bodies—to those we perceive as being in the know.

Yet, every human being is capable of error. Dr. Vinita Parkash, a professor at Yale School of Medicine, explains that as discovery within the medical industry grows more complex, the capacity for errors increases.[16] She confesses in a transparent and reflective article:

My biggest mistake (that I know of) happened early in my practice… In this case, I missed the cancer cells on my 42-year-old patient, causing her cancer diagnosis to be delayed. She eventually died of cancer.[17]

Dr. Parkash relays that pressure on doctors to be considered quality physicians by their patients, to avoid lawsuit and disciplinary action, and even to maintain esteem amongst colleagues relies on their ability to *always* have the *correct* answers to every question.[18] Certainly, even the best in their fields are incapable of putting together such a track record. By her own confession, Dr. Parkash says, the best physician is one who "makes mistakes, acknowledges them, and learns."[19]

However, this isn't how we perceive medical professionals at all, nor would we indulge them the luxury of being so transparent—so *human*. To be certain, someone who openly acknowledges this level of acceptance of shortcomings would be targeted for lawsuits or so severely mistrusted that he or she would have no client base. Thus, they must perpetuate the idea that they have earned a place on the "all-knowing" pedestal we seem so ready to position them on. It's easy, then, to see Milgram's observations alive and well today. The image of a trustworthy physician becomes all too similar to that of a comic-book hero: a superhuman, all-knowing, never-wrong champion who can save us from ourselves. And when we find someone to fill that role, we readily relinquish authority over our health to this professional.

We see this every day for those who are pursuing healing. When a medical issue surfaces, we look for an "expert" to fix it. They're easy to find: Billboards advertise attractive professionals whose very countenances ooze capability. The "shelves" of online stores overflow with "healthy" foods and supplements that are portrayed to be miracle cures for nearly anything that ails us, and fad diets allure overweight people into the notion that a monthly membership will buy the slimmer physique they desire. Added to the mix are advertisements for pharmaceuticals, medical facilities, and surgical procedures that portray thriving, happy, eye-catching people who smile reassuringly, telling consumers they "got their life back" after buying in to the symptom-covering fix-all that we call our modern medical industry.

Such media and propaganda is damaging. It distances us from our responsibility to take an active role in managing our health. Additionally, it feeds the common train of thought that if something happens to go wrong with the body, it's easily fixed. After all, we have experts to take care of that! In the meantime, symptoms are masked, and the physician who states there is no reason for further concern becomes the authority who frees patients to resume poor health habits. And why wouldn't these "experts" have such clout in the eyes of the layperson? They are professionals—precisely the type of person, Milgram demonstrated, whom people are inclined to obey, even when it goes against their own instincts or even moral code.

I (Joe) will give you a personal example. Just before I went in for my colon surgery, my wife asked the doctor if there could be any advantage to my taking probiotics. She had begun to wonder (as I have told previously in *Timebomb*) if there was a link between my medical problems and diet. The physician answered that "no science anywhere…illustrates that probiotics do anything." He went so far as to explain that many people have their colons completely removed and live perfectly normal lives.

Then, he pulled out a brochure. I'll never forget it.

The colorful piece of media was produced to assure the patient anticipating a full colectomy (complete removal of the bowel) of the hope for an ordinary, pain-free and disease-free future. However, what really stands out in my memory are the models of post-surgical patients portrayed in the publication. One was an extremely attractive woman on the beach wearing a bikini and a colostomy bag. Another model was dressed like some sort of kickboxer or cage-fighter. Not only were these models representing patients as happily postoperational, but they were extremely physically fit, even athletic. As I stated in *Timebomb*, I was so tired of being unhealthy for such a long time that I succumbed to the propaganda.

My wife, however, wasn't so quick to embrace the message. Her instinct was talking to her, and she was listening. However, because of the acuteness of my symptoms, the exhaustion brought on by years of chasing healing and feeling as though we had run out of options, and the influence of this "knowledgeable professional," we went through with the procedure.

Later, I found that literally thousands of studies link healthy gut microbiota to overall *and* specific avenues of improved health. The doctor's statement simply wasn't true. Now, please know that I hold no ill toward this physician. He is reputed to be one of the best in his practicing state, highly acknowledged and regarded by his peers, and decorated with all the symbols of success that come with performing good practice. As I stated in *Timebomb*, if a person were to opt for a surgical removal of part of his or her body, this was definitely the right guy to see.

However, this doctor's dismissal of my wife's intuition resulted in the removal of part of my colon. I forfeited—forever—the opportunity to find a natural way to heal from that illness. This decision was influenced by his authority and the trust we placed in him, the facility, and even the innovations that lent esteem to his advice.

Whether you accept the premise that Milgram's study is worth considering, it remains a fact that most people hand over their healthcare to providers. Whether it's the allure of a quick fix promised by a model on a billboard, the convenience of allowing someone else to manage your health, or even the perception of lack of individual empowerment, the sad truth stands that, for some reason, we live in a "doctor knows best" society.

It's important to note that the onus for this problem is not on doctors. For example, in my situation, despite that the physician said there was no science to back up the concept of healing through balancing gut microbiota, he gave us an answer that followed industry standards. He was merely following protocol. This is the heart of the point I'm trying to make: The responsibility is not on doctors to take over our health—it is *on us*. Few people see a physician for wellness exams, and multitudes avoid giving thought to improving nutrition through diet or supplementation, or to taking other preventative measures. Instead, most wait *until there is a problem*, then seek help from a medical professional who is expected to provide damage control for health that has already been allowed to spiral out of control. *Then*, we look to them as authority figures and miracle workers. Ask yourself this question: How can we expect these medical professionals to care for us by reversing the series of decisions we've made that may have escalated into illness?

This way of thinking leads to further problems that subsequently hinder our well-being. For example, when we don't provide proper nourishment for our bodies or take measures to fortify our immune systems, it's inevitable that we will become ill. For many, our immediate response when we're sick is to go the doctor for antibiotics. However, these damage the gut flora, which should be made up of a balance of healthy bacteria that reside in the intestine. Over time, this harms the immune system, while offering negative bacteria and even viruses the opportunity to become stronger, causing future bouts with illness to become more severe. Additionally, antibiotics have been linked with digestive problems, fungal infections, anaphylaxis, and even kidney failure. Some studies have linked the use of these drugs to cardiovascular problems,[20] delirium or cognitive interference,[21] and even Crohn's disease.[22] Yet, it seems that every time a "bug" works its way through our communities, many people (who take no preventative or immune-fortifying steps the rest of the time) take antibiotics in search of relief. We do this to our bodies, repeatedly and without question, because it's convenient, and because a doctor tells us it's the road to wellness.

On a more severe note, many folks (such as a previous version of myself, Joe), opt to have surgery to make permanent physical alterations at the advice of these professionals. When I had the segment of my colon cut out, I was told that it was literally nothing more than storage for waste matter soon to be defecated; there was no other purpose for that section of my colon than this. After I began to recover from the surgery and seek wellness via the natural method, my continual lack of energy became a concern. As I dug for answers, I finally found that the portion of colon I sacrificed is actually the area responsible for the absorption of B-complex vitamins, which are *vital* for metabolizing incoming nutrition into energy. Without the ability to take in the B vitamins, my body struggled with a severe energy lag while my taxed adrenals attempted to fill the gap by overworking—a health conundrum that required a significant recovery time. *And*, this revelation was not unearthed until I had engaged with a natural healthcare practitioner.

Blame the Doctor?

As stated previously, we're wired to follow a certain protocol for dealing with illness: We experience symptoms (usually some type of discomfort), and eventually they become troublesome enough to compel us to look for a trusted medical professional. That person then tells us what is wrong and offers treatment (usually a pill or other medication). We follow the instructions until the prescribed time-frame has expired. Then, we go on with our lives, forgetting the symptoms as long as they don't return. However, we often fail to consider that many symptoms are precisely that—*symptoms*; they are our body's way of signaling an underlying problem. We don't realize that by the time we see a medical professional, a condition of some sort has already escalated into discomfort. Unaware of the cause of our distress, we discuss symptoms with that professional, who then then gives us precisely what we are asking for: something to grant relief.

Since many providers are often unaware of the underlying problem, they consider it a success when they can mask our discomfort and make us feel better. However, when an issue lies beneath the surface and there are no red flags, the professional has no way of knowing what the source of trouble may be—or even if there is one. Thus, when warning signs are concealed, it's assumed that the patient has been restored to optimum health. Unfortunately, the central, unaddressed difficulty often continues to manifest in varying symptoms until it worsens and emerges as a chronic disorder or illness.

Many, at this point in the conversation, shake a finger at doctors and blame them for myriad flaws. Some say they are profiteers, others accuse them of being unknowledgeable, and a further crowd states that they are uninterested in patients' well-being and don't give full disclosure about side effects of medications, etc. While professionals in any industry may display such faults, those in the medical field often receive a particularly bad rap. Unfortunately, doctors can't always see the complications beneath the surface that eventually result in sickness. Furthermore, the uptick in chronic illness, cancer, and other diseases since the mid-1990s has caused many in medicine to be overwhelmed, and they're on a hard curve to understand the epidemics at hand. For many, providing health and comfort to their patients may seem like a medical version of "whack-a-mole"—they hammer away at sporadic and seemingly disconnected symptoms that keep popping up. While some may argue that conventional doctors don't adequately address overall nutrition, it's likewise true that by the time someone seeks medical care for symptoms, the underlying issues of malnutrition and years of neglecting self-care have begun to create a complicated set of circumstances. And, many of these professionals are aware that they may have little cooperation from patients regarding lifestyle changes, preferring the quick fix of drugs.

In truth, many folks who go into medicine chose their careers because they wanted to help people. In addition, many were educated and trained in preceding decades, when the nutritional value of our food was still declining and hadn't yet bottomed out, while the practice of adding dangerous ingredients to our food was on the rise, and the need for alarm hadn't yet surfaced. In other words, they're still catching up to the dire nutritional bankruptcy most patients today are suffering.

We can see an example of this through the story of my (Joe's) daughter who, several years ago, began to suffer chronic urinary tract infections (UTIs). Our doctor at the time (a Western medical professional we greatly respected; this was before we embarked on our natural health journey) gave her repeated rounds of antibiotics (which, as previously mentioned, damages the gut flora, lowering the immune system in the long run). But each time, the UTI would return in a couple of months. As we began to explore natural healthcare, I discovered D-mannose, a natural element that comes from the soil and used to be found in our food. (Incidentally, it is likewise found in cranberries, which explains the practice of taking cranberry supplements for UTI prevention. Many who suffer chronic UTIs have found success in a D-mannose regimen, as it binds to bacteria in the bladder, disabling its ability to cling to tissue, thus causing it to be expelled in urination.)

Because of over-farming, we suffer a deficiency of this vital substance. When my wife and I began to supplement our daughter's diet with D-mannose, the infections stopped. However, when I took the supplement to the doctor we thought so highly of, she said she had never even heard of it. This type of nutritional shortage in our food creates a certain brand of sabotage to the success of today's doctors. They not only have to contend with the health epidemics that are ravaging our society, but they're also expected to offer expertise regarding all the ever-changing shortcomings of our food supply—all while diagnosing any correlation between the two. Then, they're expected to individualize this gap to every patient in order to reverse and prevent related disease patterns.

Further, physicians are often accused of being "ignorant," "money-hungry," or just plain "stupid" when they're unable to diagnose the cause of ambiguous illnesses. But these symptoms are almost always byproducts of deeper issues, often perpetuated by continued (albeit often unintentional) bad decisions. Additionally, the adaptable human body keeps on trying to stave off the onslaught, perpetually morphing its response to toxins, pollutants, sedentary lifestyles, and nutritional deficiencies. This causes a huge, ever-growing variance in physical manifestations, which is why "new" conditions, disorders, and diseases are always being discovered. Even when sophisticated equipment can pinpoint a particular illness, all that does is provide a *label*; it gives little or no insight to the central problem.

In the midst of these clashing circumstances stands the Western medical professionals. They are only human. Often, they are overwhelmed (with all the issues discussed here), and this is before the size of their caseload is even brought into the discussion. Many live on call day and night and do what they do just because they care. Frequently, they simply don't have the right tools. They follow the protocols they learned during their training (an education which, by the way, leaves them with enough debt to offset their seemingly disproportionately high salaries). Because new medical conditions keep being discovered, they must roll with an ever-evolving knowledge base.

Dr. Zach Bush is a physician who specializes in endocrinology, metabolism, and internal medicine. He has expertise in hospice and palliative care, and is the director of the M Clinic in Virginia and author of numerous articles in respected, peer-reviewed medical journal articles. He is an outspoken authority on the emerging evidence linking chemical pesticides and modern pharmaceutical practices with the current, widespread health epidemic. As for the situation facing physicians who are contending with this crisis, he explains, most doctors won't reflect on this time in terms of medical procedures, but, rather through relationships that they have made along the way. Dr. Bush describes the disillusionment doctors experience when they learn they don't have all the tools they need to provide good healthcare:

> [Physicians are] never going to tell you about the science… about the drugs. They're going to tell you about…relationships they had with their patients… [but that gets overwhelmed by the fact that] we've been given a bad tool box to take care of people…[and because of this fail] at our ability to…improve the quality of health of our patients.[23]

We believe we need to restore honor to the physicians serving our society by realizing that *they* cannot make people better. They merely respond to our symptoms—and try to alleviate them to improve our quality of life. We have to realize that while doctors are good resources, our healthcare starts in *our own* hands, long before we ever place it in the hands of professionals.

As patients, we tend to pigeonhole doctors into one of two positions:

(1) as an unquestionable authority who speaks a protocol that we must follow precisely and whom we blame when we don't get well, or, (2) as an enemy because the treatment is—for *whatever* reason—unsuccessful. But if we think this way, we're viewing these specialists in the wrong light. Doctors are resources we can turn to in our pursuit of good health. Many of us expect them to "play God," but that's a game they can *never* win.

When physicians do fail, we often blame them for being inadequate or even uncaring. The truth is, in a perfect world, the pharmaceutical industry would be restructured to make consumers more aware of the shortcomings and side effects of its products; food would be grown under the safest and healthiest of circumstances and free of dangerous ingredients; medical training would be amended to include preventative care rather than just the treatment of symptoms; and profiteering at the expense of people's health would be a thing of the past.

But this isn't the world we live in—*yet*. While we exist in the realm of obstacles like the ones we've mentioned here, it's vital that we take charge of our own *preventative* care. For those who are already sick, there is hope for reversing disease or managing your illness or condition to yield a higher quality of life. For those who are not ill, we can't stress enough the importance of becoming proactive about your health—*now*—to ensure the blessing of wellness in your future.

How Did We Get Here?

A Brief History of the Dust Bowl

Just after World War I, the development of machinery emerged as an innovative strategy for struggling farmers. With new tools on the field such as plows and tractors, approximately ninety-six million acres of newly overturned farmland were planted across Kansas, Oklahoma, Colorado, New Mexico, and Texas.[24] In 1931, these plains yielded record-breaking harvests. However, as the excess of wheat flooded the postwar market, prices dropped, diminishing profits and causing, in subsequent years, fields to be left unplanted.

In previous decades, this land had accumulated its topsoil by means of depositing winds and runoff from the Rocky Mountains. This layer had been anchored by "hardy grasses which held the soil in place in spite of the long recurrent droughts and occasional torrential rains characteristic of the region."[25] The area had been largely in its primitive state in the middle 1910s, but due to soaring wheat prices during the first World War, it had seen an increase of agricultural and cattle farming activity while at its production peak: "The acreage devoted to wheat in one part of the...region tripled between 1914 and 1919 and increased more than fifty percent more in the next decade."[26] The combination of this uptick in soil disturbance, the subsequently neglected growing fields as the wheat market declined, and the use of much of the acreage for cattle (which also contributed to erosion), the drought and constant wind that ravaged the region in the early 1930s culminated in the disaster later known as the Dust Bowl.

Winds swept loose dirt, mercilessly flinging it about the land. Dry, rainless weather allowed no natural grass or other vegetation to take root and harness the topsoil. Many places, under a sky darkened by the density of these particles, lost the first three to four inches, and in some areas, entire buildings were buried beneath the aimlessly whisked-about earth, which created silt dunes standing as tall as ten feet.[27] What had begun as a seemingly prosperous and lucrative way of increasing profits and providing plentiful foods through agriculture had ended in disaster—costing thousands of families their farms and sending two-thirds of them to the West in search of a new habitat.[28]

With a very sad and expensive (on many levels) lesson on the dangers of poor farming practices apparently learned, federal, state, and local agricultural efforts increased in subsequent years to implement soil restoration. Some of these included large-scale grass seeding; timed rotations of crops such as fallow, wheat, and sorghum; the insertion of "wind breaks" built by tall, extended fencing or even rows of trees; and the promotion of techniques such as strip planting, terracing, and contour plowing.[29]

As rains mercifully began to fall again in the late 1930s, the region slowly recovered, but many remembered the brutal and unforeseen expense of these unvetted farming techniques. With the years of the Dust Bowl behind us, a new, nefarious farming bungle was about to collide with agriculture on American soil, one even more devastating than that of those years in the 1930s.

The new crisis would be the innovation of chemical farming.

The Chemical Comparison

In the years after World War II, the booming industry of petroleum was lauded as a key in the victory of the war: "Thanks to a combined effort of the government and industry, two pipelines were constructed to carry oil from Texas to Midwest and East Coast refineries…and win the war."[30] The end of WWII, however, brought a decline in demand and thus a surplus to the newfound industry, and those seeking its uses began to develop chemical agricultural treatments. For those still recovering from the Dust Bowl, these aids provided welcome relief. After all, if weeds and crops could be sprayed, then it wouldn't be necessary to till the ground as often or even rotate crops.

But, similar to the time before the Dust Bowl, farmers weren't aware of the risks involved in these new methods. Sadly, however, unlike the issues contributing to the Dust Bowl, chemical farming innovations aren't as easily reversed. These compounds are dangerous in the sense that they *attack* the food they're sprayed on, causing side effects such as "chemical leaf scorch."[31] They are devastatingly toxic to the soil: For example, one application of a popular glyphosate-based herbicide is known to kill 50 percent of the earthworms in the soil.[32] (This is disturbing because earthworms are vital to the health of the soil.) The hazardous consequences of using these chemicals has created the need to come up with new, replacement, or even complementary substances to counterattack the damage. Accordingly, the overall reliance on these toxins has perpetually increased.

Eventually, a "chemical codependency"[33] grew among these materials. Worst of all, many of these elements (often herbicides) have an antibiotic, enzyme-blocking property, which kills many of the nutrients and essential enzymes in the crop—in addition to increasing human exposure to such chemicals through consumption. Thus, we grow and eat foods that are biologically incapable of nourishing us and that carry agents that harm our health.

It seems like the dominoes just keep falling: As a result of overexposure to the chemicals, chronic soil acidification becomes a concern, because it marks the death of organic matter in the ground being farmed. Topsoil degenerates and eventually decreases, contributing to diminished nutrients, vitamin and mineral depletion, and overall smaller crops.[34] To counter the lower yields caused by these plant-attacking toxins, chemical fertilizers are then applied in an effort to restore the visible appearance of bounty to these harvests (in other words, the fruits and vegetables *appear* bigger and more appetizing). However, these fertilizers—growth-promoting substances—pose many of the same risks as herbicides: They cause added damage to the soil. Further, most of them are NPK (nitrogen, phosphorous, and potassium) fertilizers, which help the plants physically grow in depleted soil, but yield a product that seems healthy but has little to no actual nutrients.

Then the Rains Come…

In addition to these toxins creating a devastating decrease in the quality of our edible crops, a vast majority of the chemicals are water soluble, meaning that when rainfall hits them, they become part of the ecosystem when they're carried into groundwater and all permeable surfaces. They then evaporate into our cloud cover and linger in the air, ready to be carried back down by more rainfall to recontaminate the earth below, impacting the air we breathe and even indirectly affecting crops in areas that weren't sprayed with these chemicals.[35] Additionally, applying too much fertilizer constitutes a "greater amount…than the plants can readily absorb… [causing] excess greenhouse gases trapped in the atmosphere…[which likely contribute to] the increase of land and ocean surface temperatures."[36]

Antibiotic Properties Released Via Large-Scale Farming

The human body's exposure to such toxins over time contributes to cancer, chronic illness, autoimmune disease, and neurological disorders. They have the power to cross the blood-brain barrier—a protective membrane that surrounds the brain and prevents hazardous elements in the bloodstream from affecting brain chemistry.[37] Since such a high volume of poisons use enzyme-blocking properties, our bodies are under constant exposure to what is essentially antibiotic activity. This disturbs the body's bacterial genome, which is directly linked to wellness and immune system. Many of these intruders directly compromise the gut lining, the blood-brain barrier, blood vessels, and the kidney's protective systems, and can even result in neurological injury.[38]

Additionally, by stripping the nutrients from our food, we deny the body what it needs to fight disease. Often, then, the onset of illness facilitates a need for drugs—which the medical field will create and then sell at a high profit. For example, Dr. Zach Bush explains his opinion that vincristine, currently one of the most commonly used chemotherapy drugs, is constructed of an alkaloid that is naturally occurring and *should* be found in our food:

We've literally subtracted out of our food chain this…[natural alternative to] chemotherapy…[and if this substance were still in our food today, a person would have] a constant, low-grade, non-toxic, available vincristine that would be bathing the cells [of the body and warding off cancer].[39]

Instead, the body is deprived of this advantage, and the pharmaceutical industry has created the drug, which Bush states sells for $28 thousand per gram.[40]

The same way that poor farming techniques opened the curtain for the Dust Bowl and created a desolate farmland deplete of topsoil, which fostered silt dunes burying houses, barns, and cars in flying dust, the chemical practices that followed have ravaged the land in myriad subtle but deadly ways. Bank accounts are buried in debt as medications cause families to become bankrupt, chemicals fly without harness through the air and collect in areas they were never invited, and the ground from which we pull our food is depleted, toxic, and exhausted. The ecosystem is compromised, and human health epidemics have hit crisis levels.

We are now experiencing the Chemical Dust Bowl.

Food: The Heart of Our Culture

For many of us, food is a central point of culture. It's a huge indicator of our attitude toward life in general, and fills many needs beyond simple hunger, such as comfort, nurture, companionship, entertainment, celebrations, and even family bonding. It also weakens us; we sometimes use it as a substitute for emotional well-being, as a nursemaid after a painful loss, and for stirring up excitement in a sedentary lifestyle. It embodies everything from the restraint of rigidity to the indulgence of fleshly desire. Yet, as wired as we are to embrace food for extranutritional needs, we are by and large completely removed from its origin and production. On one hand, society seems to literally revolve around food; and on the other, we have no control whatsoever regarding its quality or supply. A myth related to this principle suggests that our physical appearance is a mirror of our attempts to make healthy decisions, but, as you're likely aware, many who *appear* healthy can easily have known—or unknown—health complications behind that illusion of wellness.

Separating the notion of food from culture is impossible; it will never happen. The intricacies that intertwine the two go back to the very first story of man and woman in the Garden of Eden. Unfortunately, the ties linking it to our demise trace that far back as well. Thus, our challenge cannot be to attempt to divorce sustenance from what makes us human; our quest becomes meeting food on a level that makes it *always* friend and *never* foe.

As a culture, our view of food has skewed to the point that we expect it to compensate for more than physical nourishment. We're wired to desire excitement, fulfilment, community, and even love. Because we live in a busy society where, for many individuals, these needs go unmet, we subliminally transmit these desires to our food. This concept was discussed at length in *Timebomb*:

> ...the most dangerous ingredient in our food is our attitude toward it. When that changes, we can begin to make prog-ress [toward better health]... Part of the solution [to changing dietary habits, and ultimately our health] is to face the fact that we have been seduced over time by complacency, exhaustion, and the urge for convenience in a world that keeps us busy. But, there's another angle we need to explore.
>
> Food is not emotional, nor is it entertaining. Advertising is...
>
> We want *food* to make us *feel better*. We want food to supplement the satisfaction we're not getting from a dead-end job or the fun missing in a lackluster social life. Worst of all,

the food is making us feel *worse*…. On top of that, when we gain weight because of the choices we're making, many of us withdraw [communally], keeping further to ourselves…and that feeds into our disappointment with our social lives which lowers our performance at work. See the cycle? It's only one of many wrapped up in the complicated subject of our food.[41]

Emotional Eating Destroys Health

Because we place so much emphasis upon food to meet needs aside from nutrition, we set up our diets for failure. No substance in our lives apart from God, family, and friends can fulfill the emotional needs we expect from food. The disappointment we feel when it doesn't satisfy our emotional needs often causes us to form bad habits such as overeating or even developing food addiction. This, combined with the diminished nutritional value offered by food in recent decades, has contributed to a critical state of health for the average American. An example from *Timebomb* reveals how sugar alone has contributed to the medical crises:

> In 1822, the average American consumed 45 grams of sugar every five days[42]…the amount [now found] in one soft drink… [was at that time] consumed over the period approaching a week. In 2012, the average American consumed 756 grams of sugar over the course of five days.[43] This is nearly seventeen times the amount…that we consumed in the year 1822, equaling approximately 130 pounds of sugar per individual each year!
>
> The problem is exacerbated by the fact that many of us live sedentary lifestyles, while simultaneously consuming… increasingly excessive amounts of sugar…[which is taken in] and is not burned as energy and the…[body] cannot keep up with the constant incoming supply. As sugar is ingested, the

pancreas releases insulin to attempt to deal with the…over-abundance of sugar…introduced…to the bloodstream (an occurrence during most American meals today). The pancreas responds by releasing too much insulin in an effort… to restore balance. But…by the time the pancreas receives the signal that it can stop producing insulin, it has already overproduced, resulting in a crash…[which we respond to by eating] a sugary snack as a "boost"…[perpetuating the] erratic, roller-coaster style pattern…that eventually trains our body to malfunction…resulting in the development of diabetes.[44]

Understanding Homeostasis

Homeostasis, in nearly every way vital to our health, refers to the body's state of overall management, pertaining to generating and storing energy, regulating temperature, and keeping vital functions stable. This system balances glucose and other necessary substances within the blood, and keeps such processes as blood pressure where they should be. David A Kessler, MD, author of *The End of Overeating*, explains: "It's a highly sophisticated system that can be explained simply: Many parts of the body talk to one another."[45] When the body maintains homeostasis, we can count on all systems functioning properly, with regulated eating patterns, body temperature registering between 97.7—99.5 degrees Fahrenheit, the digestive system reliably processing food and expelling waste, and sleep patterns remaining on cycle. These are the bodily functions we take for granted, and they are all a product of unwavering homeostasis.

One of the problems with chronic overeating (a regular occurrence in society today) is that the urges don't simply follow the signals sent via the homeostasis communication routes that trigger hunger prompts when the body requires calories. Instead, science shows that the body is no longer communicating honestly with itself regarding input and output.

Only in recent years has it become apparent to what extent people have been damaging their bodies by eating for entertainment or emotional reasons—a dilemma Kessler calls the "reward system"—and only now is information showing how dangerous this escalation is. It would appear that the body would regulate itself to take in less food as we become more sedentary, but this logic fails to consider the "food seduction" that occurs through the body's emotional and chemical addiction to food, either through habit, addictive ingredients, or both.

Thus, by adopting poor habits where food is concerned, we throw off our body's homeostasis and thus interrupt the flow of communications and operations between our physiological systems. This leaves us vulnerable to nearly every kind of disease, and often, it lies at the root of illness as well. (More on this later; for now, suffice to say that changing our perspective of food is one of the first steps in the direction of better health.)

A Countercultural Look at Food

We realize that many of you are aware of and have already either addressed, or are currently addressing, your own poor practices regarding food, if you have any. Because of this, we won't dwell much longer on the subject, which was covered at length in *Timebomb*. For those looking to free themselves from food addiction, it would seem that food is both everywhere and in everything. It's an integral part of weddings, birthdays, holidays, good days, bad days, celebrations, and losses. Thus, it is deeply tied to emotions. As a result, we're often defensive of our food choices and habits.

According to Dr. David Kessler, the first step toward healthier eating habits is breaking our current model of the reward system. *We must find rewards that replace food.* It's definitely a challenge: Food fills our stomachs, it tastes really good, and it relaxes us. We need to take it in regularly, and we encounter it several times daily—even when it's others who are eating or snacking. No other bad habit or addiction requires us to remain so close to what we want to free ourselves from. On the contrary, all other compulsions can be remedied by permanently removing the culprit. In our culture, however, food always lingers in the periphery, remaining as our entertainment and our comfort; always present at the highest and lowest points of our existence; and serving as the centerpiece of our family and community gatherings. Further, think about it: Eating food involves all five of our senses, which makes it hard to find a substitute. This means what when gratuitous and recreational food is removed from the equation, many of us feel completely lost. As a society, we have "lost track of what we needed to feel satisfied."[46]

The Heart of This Book

Beyond the widespread issues of overeating or disease, the heartbeat of this book, as we've emphasized, is set to empower you to take a proactive stance on behalf of your own health, because it is your birthright as a child of God to enjoy an abundant and healthy life. We wish to let you know what you can use to fight against illness, chronic disease, addiction, pain, discomfort, or *any other problem* that inhibits your ability to live a quality life.

Many who have been diagnosed with an imbalance of some sort may feel that they are without hope for improving their situation. It is vital to remember that often, even when a doctor says a condition is normal or even hereditary, reversal or quality-of-life management is very possible with the right knowledge and discipline. For those who feel they're doomed to wear the label of a diagnosis or who have felt confined to treatments only available within traditional Western medicine, a holistic viewpoint very likely will reveal that many diseases are actually *imbalances* that can be corrected with proper nutrition and lifestyle.

As you take in the upcoming pages, it is our prayer that the information, hope, and inspiration we provide will give you the power to take charge of your pursuit, leading you to achieve healing on a level you never thought possible.

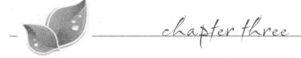

chapter three

Don't Become the Label

For as he thinketh in his heart, so is he…
~Proverbs 23:7

For many who are diagnosed with an illness, the first response—whether they realize they're doing it or not—is to embrace the label of that illness and pursue it, aligning it with their identity. For many, this means channeling resources into finding treatment or even a cure, and for others, it can even involve feeling victimized by the implications of the condition.

To use a simple example, a woman told that she has strep throat will likely be prescribed an antibiotic. It's highly likely that the very next stop she makes, after seeing her doctor, will be at the pharmacy for her medicine. She then puts upcoming activities or appointments on hold until her health has improved enough to resume daily life. Temporarily, that illness takes over her time, resources, and focus. A more serious version of this takes place when, for example, a man learns he has cancer. Usually, he will immediately begin chemotherapy or another treatment regimen mapped out by the physician. Somewhere between these two extremes another man, who is diagnosed with a manageable but chronic illness he will have to deal with for the rest of his life. For him, the coming days, months, and even years or decades can be spent marked by his search for relief. If he, like the woman diagnosed with strep throat, places other activities or engagements on hold until his good health returns before resuming normality, the result could be that his life will slowly be taken over by his illness, with anything that brings joy postponed until he feels good again. Sadly, for those with long-term or chronic illnesses, people may find themselves, years later, having completely given up the things they once only meant to place on hold, and that, while they were pursuing wellness, their quality of life dropped significantly as their sickness took over.

When we receive a name for an ailment, we often fuse that name into our own identity: I "*have* fibromyalgia" or I "*am* diabetic." Often, because we unquestioningly accept what experts (doctors, physicians, surgeons, or other medical staff) say, there is a sad acceptance of diagnoses we allow to invade our expectations of future quality of life. Well-meaning medical professionals, in an attempt to provide information, may even tell us what to expect moving forward. This can be both good and bad for those who have become ill.

For example, in my (Joe's) situation, I was initially diagnosed with diverticulitis (a painful infection found within polyps that develop in the lining of the intestine) years ago. That doctor told me that when a third flare-up occurred, it would be time to have a surgery to remove part of my colon. Again, I asked him what caused the illness and if anything could be done to prevent its escalation. His response was that the condition was probably genetic and that I could take fiber to potentially buy some time. From that moment on, over the next six years, each eruption I endured became a check-off event on a terrible countdown. Sure enough, by the time I experienced the third episode, a surgeon *did* deem me to be a strong candidate for colon surgery to remove sixteen inches of my large intestine.

What if that first doctor had focused on positive steps I could have taken to *prevent* further episodes rather than telling me of impending outbreaks and surgeries? Of course, his response was partially due to the disconnect between the medical realm of health and wellness and the natural/nutritional angle, which *does address* such concepts. But my point is, until then, I had never been told that I had a disease or ailment that couldn't be cured. The information I got in that moment slanted toward the negative future I had to look forward to and offered me no power or pathway for proactive action. It was like being told to wait for further victimization. The verdict of my "needing surgery someday," handed to me by someone I perceived to have authority, contributed to why I had little faith at first that natural options could be helpful.

If, instead, I had been given positive tools for redirecting my health at such early stages in my illness, it's likely I never even would have needed the procedure. With the right natural intervention early on, it's probable that I wouldn't have suffered subsequent illness at all. Now, allow me to be abundantly clear: I'm *not* saying that everyone who receives a diagnosis can free themselves of all successive disease just by being proactive. Such a statement would be an insult to those who are suffering from devastating or terminal medical conditions. I *am* trying to say that many diseases stem from imbalances that, if handled appropriately early on, likely wouldn't escalate to their advanced stages.

When we're told to *expect* certain negative outcomes rather than how to *prevent* them, we're disempowered in the same moment that we're diagnosed, and the sad result is acceptance. We embrace our illness and its fusion with our identity.

Diagnosis: A Road Map, Not a Blueprint

When we look at a road map, we take an aerial view of where we are in relationship to our destination. We can assess a variety of routes that connect the two points. If one road is closed, charges expensive tolls, or is even just too long and winding, we can alter our route, with the target always in sight. When using blueprints, however, we have no such liberty. The builder *must* follow the plans directly, or the result could manifest in such nonsensical features as a bathtub in the middle of a living room floor or a toilet mounted to a wall.

When considering treatment for an illness, it's important to bear in mind that while the process could be compared to looking at a road map, likening it to a blueprint could be discouraging and defeating. For example, one person may find that the methods effective for him or her aren't the same as those highly recommended by others who have been through it. Similarly, treatments some people consider ineffective may be greatly successful for others. We must learn to evaluate the success of a treatment gradually, with an eye on overall progress. It is crucial *not* to place all of our faith in an unwavering regimen merely because it has been mandated as the "best" by someone else.

It's also important to remember that we are holistic beings—we're more than ones who do or do not have an illness. A medical diagnosis is a label of coordinated data (such as information about our symptoms, lab results, etc.) that is analyzed by a physician. The diagnosis is given to us as a road map in order to help us understand the big picture of our body's struggle. From this, we can determine the general direction we need to be moving. Some people will have more options than others at this phase. For example, diabetes is related to the body's pancreatic responses to sugar and the breakdown of accurate insulin disbursement that takes place as a response. Therefore, a person diagnosed with diabetes doesn't need to say "I am diabetic" as though it's a life-long sentence, nor is that person without options for how to proceed. Rather than feeling trapped, the individual could instead say, "I need to pinpoint the cause of this malfunction and discover how to reteach my body's system." Thus, he or she can try to find the sugar-imbalance culprit (which, for many, is found in diet) and then try to correct the issue. For others (potentially those with type 1 diabetes), the options may be fewer. For those who choose to try to adjust their diet before they turn to pharmaceuticals, this doesn't mean that with the correct nutrition they'll never have an insulin imbalance again, but it *could* mean that they can live without being consumed with worry over "being a diabetic."

Many times, this road map is marked with symptoms and, as mentioned before, other physiological data. As mentioned previously, the diagnosis is almost never an actual blueprint that's set in stone or unchangeable. Usually, it's just a starting point. It's helpful to view it as a map for how to manage the dysfunction, using available knowledge as a compass for traveling in the right direction and considering the many roads and routes along the way as *individualized* opportunities for finding wellness. The diagnosis should *never* be taken personally or embraced as part of our identity. (Easier said than done, we know!) We should take the information as merely that, while rejecting the stigma that the illness brings with it.

You may indeed have an illness or disease, but bear in mind that your body was also created with the ability to heal. For some diseases, the outcomes may be more consistent with what a physician will tell you to expect, but remember: *You* are unique, and regardless of how hopeless you may feel at times, *you do not know the outcome yet*. Your body will do everything within its power not to give up on you! Additionally, faith gives us courage. In moments filled with doubt and fear, faith is made of the very things we need: It is "the *substance* of things hoped for, the *evidence* of things not seen" (Hebrews 11:1). Do you feel like you need a miracle? Then understand that faith is a valuable weapon in your arsenal! A great example of this is the placebo effect: an intangible and incalculable medical anomaly wherein those who believe they have received intervention actually manifest symptoms as though the intervention has been literally received, providing "concrete evidence that the body holds within it innate self-repair mechanisms that can make unthinkable things happen."[47]

When we believe, we know two things: 1) that we have what we need to endure, and 2) that God will continue to bestow upon us power and ability that defy our current understanding or reason.

Fight-or-Flight Response

Your brain has the power to dispatch resources toward mere survival or toward healing. It's likely that you've heard of the fight-or-flight response that takes place within the human body and mind. This is a chain reaction of physical, hormonal, and chemical responses triggered for endurance, which initiate in reaction to perceived threat. Often, those experiencing the flight response don't take the time to think rationally; they're so driven by fear that they don't think through their actions. In this moment, it's possible they'll take actions they later regret, don't remember, or even perhaps can't explain. This is because fear is the destroyer of reason. Additionally, in these moments, hormones are deployed as a means of survival. I (Daniel) have often said that when people panic, their brains can't tell what type of crisis they're facing. The brain only knows the chemical/hormonal response it's experiencing at that moment. On this level, it is merely reading data based on instinctive switches being flipped—much like an indiscriminate light switch. The setting is either "on" or "off," and the mind is unable to distinguish whether a person is being eaten by a bear or is panicking because he or she can't pay the rent. The brain only knows that hormones are being deployed and alarm is taking place. This type of hype has negative consequences on the body over time, and allowing stress to run rampant within one's thoughts contributes great overall damage to health *and* the ability to heal. Thus, as the brain recurrently deploys survival resources rather than healing resources, systems are overworked without any positive progress taking place within the body.

Additionally, when we anticipate negative events, we are, in the same way, chemically and hormonally requiring the body to live through disasters that haven't yet occurred. For example, if you are afraid you might lose your job and you ruminate on this possibility, your body must endure the metaphysical stress of that event multiple times—not just on the day it finally happens. By allowing our minds to wander to negative possibilities, we force our bodies to endure the stress response of one event over and over. (Reliving traumatic memories can trigger the same type of physical damage in this way.) Further, when we give ourselves to worrisome thoughts, we fill our extra space with this negativity rather than leaving that space for God (remember this key point for now; we'll explain further in an upcoming chapter).

When we keep fear, anxiety, and stress at bay and instead shift our thoughts to a positive direction, we begin to do something that I (Daniel) call "living strength." This literally causes a metaphysical response within the body to dispatch healing power, because the mind has chosen to deploy healing resources toward what we have decided by faith is real. I (Joe) used to have a friend who rightly believed in speaking the name of Jesus over every situation. When a person would say, "I have <insert illness here>," she would lovingly correct them by saying "You mean, 'I am fighting to claim victory over <insert illness here> in the name of Jesus.'" Neither statement denies the struggle of the illness, but one calls the individual's mind to keep faith and hope alive, while the other approach victimizes the patient and hands triumph over to illness in a battle that is not yet over.

Matthew 18:18–19 tells us that what is bound on earth is bound in Heaven, and that which is loosed on earth is loosed in Heaven. Many prosperity preachers have taken this verse out of context over the years, stating that if we desire material wealth, then to merely claim it is the first step. However, this verse isn't talking about the things this world will pursue. It is explaining that our words have the power to dispatch heavenly forces on our behalf.

Physicians, as stated previously, are not our enemies. Their diagnoses of our illnesses are valuable for our treatment. In no way are we stating that we should disregard medical advice. Rather, we need to understand that when one of the professionals places a label on our illness, that label comes from symptom analysis, categorization, and standard treatments that are often designed to make us believe we are better when discomfort subsides. However, often, doctors present worst-case scenarios an attempt to educate us. This can incite health-damaging fear within the already-sick body. During these times, we must recall the road map of options ahead of us and remember that our Creator designed our bodies to heal.

We see this very point demonstrated when we consider obesity, which contributes to many life-threatening diseases and, left unchecked, can manifest in countless forms of danger. However, those who are obese can consider multiple options for correcting the issue. They can choose to exercise, change to a more active lifestyle, opt for nutrition-based methods, join accountability groups, or seek even more extreme measures for getting the problem under control, and can begin to lose weight and gain muscle. Before long, this metamorphosis becomes apparent to all who know those who have lost weight. Over time, they may not be easily recognized by those who haven't seen them in a while. They may appear younger or more vibrant, and even subtle changes such as healthier hair and skin might be noticed. For many who have made this transformation, friends and family agree that they look much younger as thinner, yet older people than they did while they were obese in their earlier years. Changes such as this take place because our bodies are wired to thrive at every opportunity, which is why it is incumbent upon us to embody positive thoughts at all times. It is the *doing* of proactive steps that benefits our health, not the *knowing*.

The point we're making bears repeating. When we receive a diagnosis, it is vital to use the label as a tool for managing the dysfunction without buying into the stigmas that might come with it. By holding fear at bay and living with strength, we metaphysically allow our bodies to dispatch healing power. Keep a mindset that you're going to confront your health challenge by understanding that you are healing every moment you are living, because you are *designed to heal*.

Biochemical Power of Thought

Research has shown that suggestion has the power to create a metaphysical response from our bodies based on our expectancies.[48] This is known as the biochemical power of suggestion. Through this, our bodies become trained to follow " 'response expectancies'...[otherwise known as] the ways in which we anticipate our responses in various situations...[that] set us up for automatic responses that actively influence how we get to the outcome we expect."[49] Confused? Allow us to clarify.

In other words, when we believe something specific will happen with our bodies, the brain begins to dispatch resources toward generating the response we expect. Have you ever made a habit of eating certain foods together? Perhaps, for years, you ate a muffin each morning with your coffee. If you were to decide to cut bread products from your diet, you would likely find yourself wishing for that muffin at the moment you smell your coffee brewing. Or, perhaps, consider the example of someone who believes he is allergic to a certain food. He may experience a reaction, even if he were to subsequently learn that he was wrong about the allergy. Another good example of the biochemical power of suggestion can be found in a person who is normally shy but believes she is more assertive after drinking a couple of alcoholic beverages. Should her drinks be replaced with an alcohol-free cocktail, she would likely still behave in a more outgoing manner than usual because she would perceive herself to be slightly inebriated.[50]

Another example of this is illustrated by University of Texas at Austin's James Pennebaker, PhD, who stated:

If a visitor sits on your sofa and you say, "My dog has fleas," watch them start scratching. They don't have fleas, they're just paying attention differently.[51]

Pennebaker elaborates that a person's "focus of attention...ties closely to their health perceptions."[52] In other words, people can easily misinterpret symptoms as being more serious because of the anxiety that comes alongside what could be perceived to be indications of serious illness. Then, the brain's resources are allocated toward illness rather than healing. We all know of those who, at some point, have attempted to self-diagnose by consulting the Internet. Likely, they ran across the description of a serious medical illness that fit their symptoms and panicked, but, when they went to the doctor, they learned that their illness was something much less serious. However, this type of worry, over time, has the power to worsen a situation. Through the concept of biochemical power of suggestion, the body will follow the conviction of the mind.

How, on a scientific level, is this possible?

The body's endocrine system is responsible for regulating hormones, sleep, metabolism, emotional well-being, tissue maintenance and repair, and even sexual responses by sending communication throughout the body via the circulatory system. The hypothalamus gland is the connection of communication between the nervous system and the endocrine system. This means that stimulus coming into the brain is translated into messages by the hypothalamus. The messages are then disbursed throughout the body via the endocrine system, giving instruction regarding release of hormones, healing resources, heart rate and blood pressure, body temperature, and many other things, including appetite, thirst regulation, and sleep patterns.

The hypothalamus receives and relays emotional signals, including those pertaining to fear, anger, stress, or anxiety. As discussed previously, this is how the brain is able to trigger survival reactions throughout the body, such as cueing the "tingling" sensation in arms and legs as a result of the fight-or-flight response, the indication that the limbs are prepared to take swift, self-preserving action if necessary. This shows that the signal of threat is instantly regarded throughout the body, which immediately responds. This is a technique our brains have become equipped with over centuries of surviving, and it is facilitated by the hypothalamus gland.

Unfortunately, our brains seem hardwired for negative thought. This, in psychology, is a principle known as "negativity bias"—"our tendency not only to register negative stimuli more readily [than positive ones] but also to dwell on these events."[53] This is a statistically quantifiable phenomenon, meaning many studies have shown that people tend to cling to negative outcomes or feedback, and an equal amount of positive outcomes or feedback doesn't effectively offset the damage done by the destructive. (You may have heard the adage that we need to hear seven compliments for every single insult before the damage of the hurtful comment is repaired.) This is why a bad first impression can sour a relationship for a lifetime, why childhood verbal abuse can cause an adulthood of inner struggle, and why traumatic memories can be so easily relived, despite even years of healing therapy.[54] Many researchers theorize that this trait has evolved in the human mind for centuries for purposes of survival. When a predator was near, a pitfall existed, or an ingested plant caused illness, our predecessors were "programmed" to prioritize this recollection. It is the mind's built-in alert system that initiates self-preservation.

Because the brain is wired to recall negative input with more stubbornness than it does the positive, and since the hypothalamus acts in response to environmental stimuli, the intake of information in a particular setting can create long-lasting habitual recall. For example, a factor associated with traumatic events—such as a location, sound, voice, scent, or physical touch—can act as a trigger, causing someone to chemically relive dire events for years after the fact. On the other hand, a song associated with a happy time can bring back a memory of carefree, youthful days, and the smell of a flower can recall one's thoughts to a beautiful summer vacation long ago.

The good news is that our minds can be retrained. The application of this principle is much easier said than done, but by forcing negative thought patterns out of our minds and embracing positive, hopeful ones, we mandate the brain to create a new habit. At first, this is difficult.; recall that the negativity bias insists that we cling to what can go wrong, rather than to what is good or right. However, the more regularly we make positivity a habit, the easier it becomes, yielding emotional, chemical, and physical benefits.

We've mentioned that the hypothalamus communicates foreboding emotions such as anger, fear, stress, or anxiety. However, it's interesting to note that the hypothalamus is also responsible for the nervous tension that, once accompanied by such "feel-good" hormones as dopamine, oxytocin, and vasopressin (each of which is also initiated by the hypothalamus), develops into friendship, affection, and even romantic sensations such as love.[55] This makes sense when we recall the "butterflies in the stomach" feelings of initial attraction—that mix of anxiety and thrill. Because dopamine is one of the body's biological rewards, the compulsion to return to the person who triggers such a response within us eventually becomes strong enough to help a friendship (or incidental meeting) grow into love.[56] When oxytocin is initiated through the hypothalamus, it's usually accompanied by the sensation of physical touch. Vasopressin solidifies relationships by contributing to affectionate feelings that foster "social bonding with a partner."[57]

Because of the hypothalamus' role in the emotional part of our brain, coupled with its efficacy as communicator to the endocrine system, we can easily see how our mood impacts the chemical responses dispatched throughout our entire bodies. This shows that the brain has a literal, physical connection to our emotional well-being and our bodily functions.

Many people confess they've noticed a link between their mood and their appetite, energy level, libido, ability to obtain a good night's sleep, or even fight illness. These are all related to the communications sent throughout the endocrine system via the hypothalamus. In addition, as noted earlier, it's an unfortunate fact that the brain is wired to hang on negative thoughts with more stubbornness than its willingness to embrace positive ones. However, when the mind is filled with positivity, we can see the chemical link between these thought patterns and overall health. This impacts the immune system, the functionality of vital organs, circulation, metabolic processes, cardiovascular activity, sleep, reproductive health, and much more. Likewise, even active physical responses such as affectionate and passionate touch are influenced, which, in turn, impacts our relationships. In this way, we act out our thoughts, which feed our state of mind, perpetuating our health in cyclical fashion. The brain, via the hypothalamus gland, literally has the power to dispatch the damaging fight-or-flight response discussed previously, or it can send healing resources through the body that keep systems balanced, regulated, and functioning at optimum levels for maximum health.

It's a liberating and thrilling thought to realize that we have vast influence over our health just by regulating our thoughts.

What If It's Hereditary?

The genetic lineup you inherited from your parents is not the same as the one they received from their parents, since gene expression changes according to what the body is currently doing. Thus, the decisions we make today literally cause our DNA to adapt. We previously discussed those who, after fighting obesity, appear younger and healthier in subsequent years than they did previously, despite the fact that they have become older. At the level of genetic expression, this is also true. The lifestyle choices we make affect us all the way down to the cellular and genetic levels (this will be covered at more length in an upcoming chapter).

Many are surprised to learn that our genes began in our grandparents.

The decisions they made, the foods they ate, their level of activity, and even their chemical exposures or consumptions shaped the DNA they handed down to their children—our parents. Then, the lives of our own parents contributed further to shaping these factors through the same elements: food, lifestyle, activity, etc. Some elements aren't as easily controlled, such as exposure to pollutants or sunlight and fresh air, which can derive from one's regional situation or employment setting. However, the DNA our ancestors nurtured and passed to us is the genetic heritage we receive. In turn, we handle this precious commodity for a while in our own bodies before passing it on to our children. As we live and make decisions, our genetic genome continues to change and update according to the way we live and everything we expose our bodies to. Then, we hand this down to our own children.

This is both very good and very, very bad. Many people eat the way that they want with the assumption that *they* are the only one they might be hurting. This is wrong if there are children in their future. When people allow their bodies to be exposed to excessive chemicals or poor nutrition, or if they indulge in using illegal drugs, excessive alcohol, or tobacco, they are placing telltale marks on the genome that will become part of their children's inheritance. The good news, however, is this: Over the course of our lifetime, we are each rewriting our own DNA. We have the power to strengthen our children's ability to live long and healthy lives.

When we make good decisions, our resilience improves. This is why someone who is inactive or obese can make a decision for better health and experience an empowering physical overhaul just by changing diet and activity. It is, of course, hard at first, but by starting healthier habits, he or she is rewarded with a literal, *physical* change. If you decide you want a more muscular physique, you can begin to work specific muscles, and the body will undergo a metaphysical realignment. Your BMI (body-mass index) will improve, fat percentage will decline, and lean tissue will bulk up. In a different way, you can decide to make healthier dietary choices, and eventually, your taste buds will begin to crave healthier foods. (We've all probably known someone who notes such a difference following an intentional change in lifestyle). As a result, "hereditary" inclinations such as being predisposed to obesity or diabetes will begin to realign genetically, allowing you and even your future children better health. We can't emphasize enough that it is your responsibility to make wise decisions with your body, because you are *literally* constructing the genes that will be building blocks for the next two generations.

In my (Joe's) previous work, *Timebomb,* we discussed how dangerous food ingredients impact the genetic makeup of future generations:

> [Often,] people don't know…that our DNA can adapt to the dietary changes we implement in our own bodies. These changes can then be inherited by our children. Dr. Mercola made this alarming statement about the possibility that what we're eating will cause our children to suffer:

> > It's now well known that dietary changes can prompt epigenetic DNA changes that can be passed on to future generations. For instance, pregnant rats fed a fatty diet had daughters and granddaughters with a greater risk of breast cancer. It could be that we are just now starting to see these types of generational effects showing up in humans, caused by our grandparents' and parents' penchant for processed foods. If that's the case, then we have even more incentive to make drastic changes, and soon, because the disease trends we are now seeing are only going to get worse as much of the processed foods consumed today are not even food based! So who knows what kind of genetic mutations and malfunctions we are creating for our future generations when a MAJORITY of our diet consists of highly processed and artificial

foods. As it stands, 90 percent of foods Americans purchase every year are processed foods![58]

Knowing that what we eat can change the physical traits we hand down to our children literally means that the health that's been granted to us is our responsibility to pay forward to our children. They deserve it, and they're counting on us for it.... It is important that we take care of our own bodies for the sake of our children and our grandchildren, yet unborn, just the same way that we would adjust the way we are feeding the ones who have already been born.[59]

In the same way many parents and grandparents strive to leave a monetary inheritance to their children, it's important not to overlook hereditary health; in fact, it is likely the more important of the two!

The Word "Terminal"

This book wouldn't be balanced if we were to ignore the likelihood that some of you (or a loved one) are diagnosed with something that a physician called "terminal." We'd be shortsighted if we didn't acknowledge the fear, vulnerability, and intimidation you face when you hear that word. Unfortunately, life is filled with questions that are difficult to answer, and the questions that pop up during times when we receive a grim diagnosis are some of them. In such situations, we pray God will grant complete and miraculous healing, while offering this book in the hopes that the information will bring the utmost quality to each forthcoming moment of life.

Often, people don't understand why when, after claiming healing in the name of Jesus, they aren't physically relieved of their pain. Maybe they even pass away. At these moments, life seems cruel and unjust, administering pain on the undeserving or innocent (especially when the patient is a child). Some even wonder if they didn't pray hard enough or show enough faith, punishing themselves for what they perceive to be a lack of miraculous intervention on God's part. Adding insult to injury are those who take the following scriptural passage out of context: "Who his own self bare our sins in his own body on the tree, that we, being dead to sins, should live unto righteousness: by whose stripes ye were healed" (1 Peter 2:24). Many times, when a loved one dies from a terminal illness, those left behind suffer the grief of feeling that healing was promised, but not delivered. Often, anger at God is an outlet for this intense pain.

We realize that this is a delicate subject, as being (or having a loved one) diagnosed with such a disease brings emotional devastation. When people look to passages such as the one from 1 Peter mentioned previously, the physical healing that does not occur leaves many wondering if God has abandoned them in their hour of need. Some comfort may be taken from the verse that immediately follows that one: "For ye were as sheep going astray; but are now returned unto the Shepherd and Bishop of your souls" (1 Peter 2:25). The second verse gives insight to the previous. The healing referenced is that of being *delivered from sin*. As sad as death is to accept in this earthly realm, it is comforting to understand that ultimate healing has been purchased by Jesus, and it is bigger than the curing of our bodies within this realm. Because of His sacrifice, we have been given restoration in *the next life: that of joining Jesus in Heaven*. We have a sure and certain hope in this healing, and we can look forward to a body that does not become ill:

> For we that are in this tabernacle [of earthly flesh] do groan, being burdened: not for that we would be unclothed [relieved of our earthly bodies], but clothed upon, that mortality might be swallowed up of life... Therefore we are always confident, knowing that, whilst we are at home in the body, we are

absent from the Lord…We are confident…and willing rather
to be absent from the body, and to be present with the Lord.
(2 Corinthians 5:4, 6, 8)

Essentially, we're explaining that while we seek a cure in this life,
those who face terminal illness often believe they must swallow the bitter
pill of exclusion from this Scripture, as though, for some reason, they
missed out on these promises. It helps to understand that these verses
explain that God has purchased us a wonderful future, but for some, the
next life comes sooner than it does for others. The most beautiful part of
our healing is that true wholeness begins when we enter the presence of
God at the end of our earthly lives. We are assured that God, Himself,
personally rights all wrongs and promises us we will never know pain or
sorrow again:

God shall wipe away all the tears from their eyes; and there
shall be no more death, neither sorrow, nor crying, neither shall
there be any more pain: for the former things are passed away.
(Revelation 21:4)

Even as we write these pages, we're praying for you, the reader,
that this book will offer hope and comfort throughout your search for
healing.

As We Move Forward

The upcoming chapters have been written to illuminate some essentials
that exist in natural creation to help our bodies align with good health.
Some of these concepts may seem overly simple at first, but they are
effective—and, better still, they're available to nearly everyone, free of
charge. What is surprising about each is that scientific information links

these elements to good health, and their deficiencies to illness. These are liberating concepts that empower us to chase well-being within our own resources, since they're accessible to everyone and are placed here as a gift from our Father in Heaven. When we really study each of these resources and see the ways that—even from a scientific standpoint—they can bestow good health on the human body, it's exciting to see that we're not captive to a certain income bracket, region, or demographic to pursue good health. God has placed it here, within His own creation, for the taking.

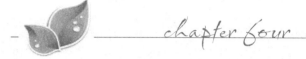

chapter four

Lifestyle and Fundamental Essentials

We have stressed the vital need to decide not to adopt the label of an illness as an identity. We've emphasized how important it is to feel empowered to shed the stigma associated with diagnoses. However, equally necessary is understanding that we don't intend to present any one supplement or regimen as a miracle cure-all. Instead, there are basic principles we can follow that will unlock the doors to greater overall wellness. Just as our bodies are made of substances from the earth, they likewise need elements from the earth to survive. When we understand that there are essentials we need to properly handle in order to obtain good health, we will find that we have much influence over maintaining vibrancy—merely by modifying our lifestyle.

These are *necessary* components for our ability to thrive. They may *appear* optional to those of us who live a busy lifestyle, but it must be emphasized that *they are not* for those who hope to enjoy optimal well-being.

Creating Space

It's highly unusual to hear anyone complain that he or she has too much time, money, or energy. In fact, quite the opposite: A vast majority of those in our society say they feel they're continually running low on these resources. Many even live out a vicious cycle that is deficient in all three areas. We need more money, so we work more. This results in a shortage of time and energy, which compromises both our physical and emotional well-being. Additionally, when we're busy and exhausted, we may then begin to pay for time-saving conveniences (such as fast food), which further compromise our overall health and don't replenish a frazzled body and mind with necessary nutrients.

I (Joe) had a friend who attended Financial Peace University courses offered by a local church, which featured American author, businessman, public speaker, and financial advisor Dave Ramsey. My friend was hoping to get good pointers on how to manage her finances, but throughout the course, found some principles that applied to life as well. She learned that we should always allocate a certain percentage of our money as a tithe or offering, and put another percentage into savings.[60] *Furthermore*, the course emphasized that if we're unable to do that, then we are living outside our means, since it's a sure thing that life *will* throw us an emergency that we won't be able to afford if our day-to-day living takes all our income to the very last penny.

This seemed reasonable, but was even more interesting when my friend told me that in studying her own finances, she had learned something new about herself: She managed her time and energy the way she handled her money. In other words, she had bills that claimed every dime of her income, leaving no room for the unexpected. In the same way, she found she had scheduled each and every moment of her day, leaving no room for the unexpected. Every day, from the minute she woke up until late at night, her time and energy were completely booked up with appointments, work, kids' soccer games, church obligations, and other commitments. There were no pockets of "free time," for simply sitting and winding down…resting, recharging. Even when she explored whether she had what many would call "me time," she found that activities she had *thought* she engaged in for personal enjoyment were really obligations.

After this reality check helped her honestly assess her practices, my friend began to eliminate things that drained her finances, her time, and her energy. As she created a "buffer zone" around her budget and her schedule, her general anxiety levels deescalated because three of her most valuable resources—her time, money, and energy—weren't always tapped to their very limits. This is a good example of a mistake that many of us make: We don't leave ourselves any reserves where issues of finances, time, and energy are concerned.

In my (Daniel's) work, one of the first things I try to teach people about altering their lifestyle is a principle I call "creating space." This applies to our time, money, energy, and anything else we feel we're running low on. When we run at break-neck speed from the moment we wake up to the instant we crash at night, we damage our health in many ways, *and* we leave ourselves no grace period for when we sense the need some down time to repair.

First of all, our bodies are not the same machine twenty-four hours a day. Throughout the cycle of a day, we're wired with surging and ebbing strengths and weaknesses, meaning we're unable to perform the same tasks with the same vitality at any point in time, on demand. We all have an internal clock called the circadian rhythm (more on this in an upcoming chapter), which dispatches certain chemicals and hormones at different times of the day. In other words, as we go about our routine activities, our bodies experience peak times for alertness and energy. Whenever we can, we should schedule business or other activities during those optimum times. Along the same note, there are lulls during this cycle when our bodies are attempting to tell us to rest. Again, if possible, it's probably a good idea not to schedule high-level activities during those "down times." It's necessary that we pay attention to these dips, because this time of inactivity allows our bodies to heal, rest, and even create and circulate chemicals and hormones that help facilitate metabolism, detox our systems, and get the vital sleep we need, among other things. For those who are constantly on the go, signals of drowsiness are the body's requests for respite. Unfortunately, we often ignore these cues or counter-attack with sugary snacks, caffeinated coffee, or worse—toxic energy drinks. Such tactics deprive us of our capability of sustaining sustain good health long-term, and they sabotage our ability to listen to what our body is saying.

One of the first steps, then, toward obtaining and maintaining good health is to learn to create space in our lives. We usually find our schedule is a great place to start.

Let me guess: You just laughed a little. Easier said than done, we know!

Creating space in our schedule usually fosters (to borrow Dave Ramsey's terminology again) a "snowball" effect that allows us to begin to relieve overcommitment in other areas as well.[61] Think about this: If you were to cut just *one* commitment each week and set aside that time for rest and silence, what would happen? First of all, the rest your body is deprived of would be somewhat recompensed. Then, the free time might find you deciding to take a walk and enjoy the outdoors, which would yield several benefits: Your body would receive vital nutrients from the sun and the outside oxygen (more on this later); it would have the opportunity to engage in invigorating and refreshing activity (again, more on this later); and you wouldn't be spending the money you might otherwise have spent had you been in the "rat race" where you've likely made it a habit to spend money. And the chain of positive events doesn't stop there. You might think about using that extra time to prepare a healthy meal at home for dinner that night rather to picking up something expensive, fast, and unhealthy. The home-cooked meal will give your body better nutrition and avoid ingredients that sabotage your health. Perhaps you might feel the energy to dig out an old board game (remember those?) and enjoy some electronic-device-free time with your family. You might seize the quiet time to pray or meditate, which have their own physical and mental health benefits (more on that in a bit), *and*, while you're in supplication or thought, you might finally receive mental clarity on an issue that's been bothering you with your family or at work.

See how this small alteration in your life can yield regularly scheduled, *extremely* beneficial fruit?

And, by applying this principle to other areas in your life, such as finances, you can improve your well-being and increase your ability to be able to set some funds aside to help with emergencies or even preventative, natural healthcare. By applying this to your energy, you're making a statement about the priority of your health. This is a hard one, because often people who mean well feel they need to carry certain torches ("If I don't do it, who will?"). Think of all the church volunteers who do as much as they do because there is a lack of other workers. This is a chronic problem, and we understand. But, in many cases, *nobody will step up* until an exhausted worker still carrying that torch finally lays it down. We simply *must* give ourselves permission to prioritize our own health. If we don't, we risk developing chronic illness, which will likely remove us from a variety of tasks anyway.

We don't just encourage you to free up space in your schedule; we believe it's vital to create space in our minds, which makes more room for God. How can we hear His voice when our thoughts are constantly running? God instructs us to wait upon Him (Psalm 27:14; Isaiah 40:31) and to listen for a still small voice, even in the wildest storms (1 Kings 19:11–13). How can this take place when we can't even stop long enough to hold one full, uninterrupted conversation with a friend? Or when we have a six-month-old stack of unread mail beside our front door. How can we hear what God is saying to us *now*?

We are far too busy, and it's wrecking our spiritual, psychological, familial, and physical health. We must learn to create space.

Creating space in our lives leaves time for joy and faith to take seed and sprout within our minds. It allows us to have peaceful intervals wherein we can develop positive thought patterns that begin to anticipate God's work in our lives. It becomes inspiring when we realize that we have a choice in whether to run ourselves ragged or realize that we have the power to put healthy boundaries around how we spend our time, money, and energy.

You may be thinking: *That sounds very well, but there is nothing I can cut!* You may believe that's true, but *surely,* you can find some way to trim back. Keeping this thought on a strictly hypothetical note, if you were to find out you had a chronic (or God forbid, even terminal) illness, what obligations would you remove from your schedule, finances, or other area of your life? Many of us *believe* we need much more than we do. Likewise, we *believe* the activities we spend our time on are much more necessary than they sometimes are.

We challenge you to start with one easy step: Look carefully at your lifestyle and determine what small adaptation you can make to achieve greater simplicity. How can you manage your time to create more space for your own well-being? One adjustment will likely have a ripple effect throughout your entire world, creating relief in other areas as well. This, like so many other statements in this book, proposes a healthy change that you can start immediately, and it likely comes free. However, the benefits will be (literally!) immeasurable in the long run, and we fervently petition that you begin to create room in your life as soon as humanly possible.

As you're evaluating how you spend your time and other resources, we ask that you assess your level of joy—an element of life that has immense influence on your well-being. Joy, in fact, is a fruit of the spirit (Galatians 5:22–23) and is like a medicine to the soul (Proverbs 17:22). If joy is lacking, try to find out why. We believe a deficiency in joy can potentially be as dangerous as the insufficiency of many essential nutrients. Because the mind is so powerful in the role of our overall wellness, it stands to reason that peace, contentment, and happiness are indispensable on our journey to good health.

Life at Home

The quality of our situation at home is another big-hitter when it comes to modifying our lifestyle to maintain good health. In 2017, the *World Happiness Report* revealed that a good balance between work and home life is "one of the strongest predictors of happiness."[62]

Didn't see that coming, did you?

Elaboration on this information shows that more than 50 percent of Americans are unhappy with their employment situations because of an improper balance between their jobs and home life, and they reportedly have little control to rectify the problem.[63] In other words, many of us are spread too thin. The "balance" ("imbalance," in this instance) refers to our ability to flexibly prioritize many universal elements of life, such as "work, family, friends, health, and personal growth." When properly balanced, these beget "a sense of purpose, belonging, and happiness."[64] Unfortunately, for the many people who feel their lives are out of such equilibrium, the powerlessness they feel perpetuates their anxiety.

We won't linger on the matter of employment, but will say that the issue is a big problem in our society, and many people carry the physical consequences in the form of anxiety, lack of sleep, or illness. Likewise, there is much to say about home life. First and foremost, our homes need to be a place of rest, shelter, and peace. As sad as it is to say, a high number of people, for one reason or another, are unhappy with their home lives. Issues such as divorce, child abuse, substance abuse, and other challenges can make one's residence a place of dread for those who dwell there. This reinforces the concept that if we are seeking to improve our health, few places serve as a more effective starting point than by insisting on peace in our homes. Such a boundary will alleviate the fight-or-flight response that so many people encounter while at home, often resulting in physical penalties. In addition to the positivity that comes with having a serene home life, the body's inflammatory system is less likely to trigger as a defense mechanism, the immune system functions more effectively, and the body's chemical and hormone emissions operate optimally. This lends to better quality and quantity of sleep, improved stress management, and an even more solid sense of familial community—all of which lead to better physical and psychological health.

Blue Zones

Research in the past decade has revealed a surprising yet liberating piece of information: Unlike what was believed in previous years of research, only 20 percent of the factors that play into the length of our lifespan is decided by our genetics. An astonishing *80 percent* of our longevity is actually determined by things like diet, activity, community interaction, atmosphere at home, access to nature, and other lifestyle factors.[65] Often, these are dictated by our environment. This research has been confirmed by studying areas in the world where people tend to live longer, healthier lives than in other regions. Citizens of these areas, known as "Blue Zones," experience, on average, half the rate of heart disease that typical Americans, are 40 percent less likely to suffer from dementia, and generally have lifespans that are approximately eight years longer than usual.[66]

Such areas include Sardinia, Italy, which boasts the highest population of male centenarians known today; and Okinawa, Japan, which hosts the largest group of centenarian females.[67] Other areas include Nicoya, Costa Rica, where the average individual is expected to live to age ninety-two, and spends "1/15 the amount of money on healthcare as North America does."[68]

Ikaria, Greece, is the Blue Zone where a man named Stamatis

Moraitis moved at age sixty-six after living in the US most of his life. He was diagnosed with cancer in 1976, and was given less than a year to live. However, he was so off-put by the exorbitant cost of funerals in America that he decided to migrate back to his homeland, Greece. He likewise decided he wanted to live his remaining time out peacefully, opting against chemotherapy treatments. To this effort, he began to spend time in his garden, and threw his energies into tending his family's vineyard. But a funny thing happened. Instead of dying that year, or the next, or *even the next*, he grew stronger. Nearly forty years later, Stamatis Moraitis finally passed away of old age in February, 2013, at the age of 102.[69]

You may be surprised to learn there is even a Blue Zone in California: the city of Loma Linda. The area is primarily populated with members of the Seventh-day Adventist faith, which forbids drinking and smoking, and encourages vegetarianism.[70] Even caffeine is off limits to those strongest in this faith, and because the religion discourages the use of *any* drugs, natural healthcare is often the first response to any ailment.

So what is it that these places have in common, creating an atmosphere where residents are able to enjoy such optimum health?

Dan Buettner coined the term "Blue Zones," in a 2005 article in *National Geographic* discussing the secrets to living a long life. Since then, Buettner has done lots of additional research, participated in speaking engagements, become a *New York Times* best-selling author, and coproduced an Emmy-winning documentary. Much of his additional research and articles reflect his attempt to identify which elements in Blue Zones are different than those in areas where people live shorter, less healthy lives. He came up with a list that includes such qualities as a community effort to reduce the availability of processed or fast foods, while making products such as fruit and vegetables more affordable and accessible. Buettner also found that the diets of those living in Blue Zones primarily consist of fruits and vegetables, with little to no meat or dairy. Physical activity is integrated into lifestyle, with many traveling by foot or bicycle rather than car. However, although these people are *on the move* more often than the average American, they're not necessarily *on the go* nearly as often, meaning, they have more leisure time for social engagement, prayer, meditation, and even napping! People who live in these zones often have strong religious roots and offer purpose to other members of their community regardless of age or ability. This fosters a situation where people feel supported by each other in a setting where their own contributions are vital. Further, family holds a place of high priority for residents of these areas.[71]

Buettner also found that a person's environment and circle of friends are huge contributors to well-being. For example, if our friends have unhealthy habits, such as smoking or drinking excessively, it is likely that we will have a hard time avoiding those activities. However, surrounding ourselves with healthy friends fosters good habits.[72]

Most exciting of all, Blue Zones can *be created*. Since Dan Buettner started his work, at least two new Blue Zones have developed. The first—North Karelia, Finland—is worth noting because, before it implemented a different communal lifestyle, it held the "highest rate of cardiovascular disease in the world."[73] An epidemiologist coordinated efforts with citizens to overhaul the area's access to and use of healthier food, and the reward was "an 80% drop in coronary mortality in middle-aged men over a 30-year span."[74] The rewards are *tangible*, and thanks to Buettner's efforts, the trend is catching on. As of 2017, thirty-one cities in America had made efforts to limit the number of fast-food restaurants, increase convenience of natural exercise through amenities such as bicycle lanes and hiking trails, and banning smoking in certain areas.[75] Regarding the concept of creating a Blue Zone in our own areas, Buettner said, "How we emulate what they do in our houses and communities can [stretch] our lifespan by 10 years."[76]

Did you catch that? You could add up to ten years to your life just by following the simple principles that are integrated into the daily lives of those who live in Blue Zones! And, if you can recruit others in your community to join you, you could see an improvement in health throughout your locale.

Most of us don't realize how vital the environment is to our physical and psychological health. Additionally, many don't realize that we spend 80 percent of our lives within a twenty-mile radius of home. This means that if our home isn't in a health-advocating community, we're likely surrounded by factors that encourage illness. This also means that it is imperative that we have everything we need in order to live a healthy life within twenty miles of our home, or we may not find ourselves with regular access to it.

For example, I (Joe) had a friend who decided to join a gym (personally, I'd rather see someone opt to exercise outdoors because of the additional benefits offered by the clean air and sunshine, but at least he was trying to improve his well-being). This friend went and worked out twice, but because he had joined an athletic club thirty-five miles from his house, he rarely "got out that way." Surely you can relate. We need all of the necessities of good health no more than twenty miles from our home. This includes a safe outdoor location for exercise, access to clean and nutritious food, good healthcare and childcare, stable employment or other wage-earning potential, accessible transportation, and valuable social/community connections.

Calculating Chronology

Many discussions about length of life include terms such as "lifespan" and "life expectancy" interchangeably. While this isn't necessarily inaccurate, each of these terms *does* refer to a specific angle of life's chronology. For clarification, these terms are defined below:

Chronological age: A person's actual age as calculated by a calendar.

Biological age: The age that physical and cognitive condition indicates when taking into account factors such as lifestyle, diet, physical fitness, and general well-being. (This is similar to the technique used for contestants in the NBC television show *The Biggest Loser*, wherein these obese individuals were told their *physical* age, which was often much older than their chronological age due to their poor fitness levels.)

Health span: The length of time a person is expected to live while enjoying good health and quality of life both physically and cognitively.

Life expectancy: A generalized estimation, usually based on statistics, of the number of years a person will live, taking into consideration demographic factors, environment, and other relevant issues.

Choices

One of the greatest forces that drives our bodies toward or away from good health is our minds—more specifically, our *choices*. Often, these are clouded because we either believe that we have no options—which is rarely the case—or we struggle to know which choices are best. Clearly, we can see from the Blue Zones that what we intentionally surround ourselves with and participate in greatly influence our health. This is both liberating and devastating: Those who see the results of previous bad decisions impacting their current health wish for a "redo" button, yet, we look ahead to realize that *we* hold a vast amount of power over where we—and our bodies—are headed.

It is essential, in my (Daniel's) view, that when we make a choice, we understand *why* we are doing so. By getting a grasp of what factors influence our decisions, we develop a conviction about the actions we take. For example, a person who gives no thought to what he or she eats may consume nearly anything that is perceived to taste good, with no further criteria impacting that selection. Once someone has resolved to try to eat healthy, a stronger element of conviction directs meal selection. This intensifies as the person begins to see pounds drop off or as he or she begins to physically feel better.

It seems that the vast majority of people navigate their lives by their own experiences or by what they personally find valuable. What we choose to prioritize becomes the fuel that reinforces our decisions, but sadly, this has a profoundly negative effect when considering those who have minimal knowledge of how the body and the environment interact. This often yields negative health consequences, and in response to diminished wellness, we tend to return to less-healthy choices in search of comfort…which perpetuates the cycle.

The first and most important decision you must make if you want to change your lifestyle is the determination to be brave. In a world where everyone seems to have an opinion, advocating for your own health can mean stepping out on our own and stating that you have chosen to pursue the avenue of health in the way your convictions lead. This may cause some backlash from those who don't agree with you. However, you are closer to your own body than anyone else can possibly be, and these people will need to trust your connection to it. While there is wisdom that should be prayerfully considered when friends and family weigh in regarding your pursuit of health, ultimately, we hope they will accept and respect your decisions.

Stress Management

As we've already touched upon, the decision to think positively enhances health in ways that are both mental and physical. In addition, sometimes keeping stress—and its impact—out of our lives must be a cognitive choice. Recall that we mentioned that the body reads all negative chemical responses in the same way: It doesn't matter if you're stressed over money or about being eaten by a bear. Thus, it is vital to keep stress to a minimum for optimal health. Yet, it seems that we are all capable of being inundated with stress if we allow this to happen. It is necessary to make an intentional effort to manage stress at all times. We can do this by eliminating the source of the problem (when possible and appropriate), praying and meditating, creating space, confiding in a comrade, or even finding activities to take our mind off the problem altogether.

Technology

Technology is a source of many joys and much pain in our modern society. It's how we keep in touch, follow local and worldwide news, pay bills, attend school, and watch movies or television programming. However, technology can be intrusive in many ways as well, and it's necessary to keep this tool in balance within our lives. Social media is a cruel tease, often only showing us what we want but don't have. Instant messages and texts can invade our private lives and create a lack of quality time with friends, loved ones, and families. Surely we've all, at some point, seen a family at a restaurant together, with each person at the table so enthralled in their phones that they didn't even speak to one another. This is another way social media robs us of community while posing as precisely that. Further, spending too much time staring at an electronic screen actually has the power to throw off our circadian rhythm (which we'll discuss in an upcoming chapter), making it difficult for the body to create chemicals that encourage vital functions such as metabolism, activity, and sleep. All in all, technology should be used as a tool when it's needed, and then set aside.

Particularly as it pertains to children, there are many health risks associated with excessive exposure to electronic devices. First, the screens put out enough amounts of blue light to interfere with the body's ability to wind down for sleep—thus fostering insomnia, which is detrimental because sleep is vital to healing, growth, and cognitive function (this will also be covered in an upcoming chapter). So, for young people whose bodies and minds are still developing, this is particularly damaging. Additionally, the blue light emitted during screen time can damage the eyes, causing them to age prematurely.[77] "It can also trigger serious conditions later in life such as age-related macular degeneration, which can lead to blindness."[78] Worst of all, the younger the eyes are that stare at the technological interface, the easier it is for the damaging properties of this type of light to be carried to the retina, meaning that the youngest viewers are most vulnerable.[79] How do parents combat this risk? By requiring children to take frequent breaks from media so that their eyes are not exposed to screens for long periods.[80]

In addition to premature aging and potential damage to the eyes, doctors cite poor posture and inactivity, over long periods of time, as extremely negative byproducts of overindulgence in sedentary lifestyle. The profits of exercise, clean air, and exposure to sunlight (discussed later) are vital components of a healthy life—especially for those still developing physically and mentally. This multitude of benefits is missed for children who spend their days lounging on a sofa and staring at a screen.

The psychological interference of digital intrusion upon the young, developing mind must not be overlooked, either. In her groundbreaking book, *Unscrambling the Millennial Paradox*, Allie Anderson reveals many ways the necessary growth of a child's psyche—even including the brain chemistry and neurological development of the mind—is inhibited by overindulgence of this pastime. While the information gleaned can easily cover hundreds of pages, for the sake of time, we will mention just a few points from that work here. To begin with, Anderson explains the science around how personal and interpersonal development are hindered by the interference of technology:

> For many people, the mass amounts of screen time that they have been subjected to literally reroutes and alters the neural pathways of the brain, impacting one's ability to connect emotionally and socially with other people, interfering with such human attributes as empathy, relatability, and contributing to isolation, depression, and an inward focus (often interpreted by others as narcissism). Beyond this, excess of digital interface

diminishes a person's ability to feel a sense of mastery or personal competence [due to feelings of inadequacy which are fostered by comparison games played over mediums such as social media], and these are detrimental losses, because it is these attributes which allow a person the courage and self-confidence to venture into purposeful life pathways, such as pursuing academic success, overcoming personal obstacles with problem-solving, critical thinking, and even taking larger risks, such as entrepreneurial endeavors or stepping out on a limb to take a professional promotion.[81]

It is easy for parents to overindulge the kids' desire for and dependence on electronics; after all, screen time seems to entertain them, keeps them occupied, and thus, seemingly keeps them out of physical danger. But few who give their children free rein in this activity stop to count the sheer number of hours children spend mesmerized by screens over the period of a week. Anderson gives shocking statistics:

Statistics show that most children begin watching television before the age of two, and between the years of 2 and 5, the typical time spent engaged in this activity is 32 hours per week. From 6 to 11 years old, the reported allotment drops to 28 hours per week. Of this activity, 97% of viewing is spent watching live TV. Beyond this, 71% of children between 8 to 18 years of age are stated to have a TV in their bedroom, and likewise spend an average of 1.5 hours more than those who do not have a private television. As a result, those who spend the most time engaging in this activity also often do so in isolation and without supervision or parental filter. Furthermore, two-thirds of households report leaving television sets on while eating meals, substituting interaction with one's family for a digital interface.[82] The danger that this activity poses surfaces over time and on many levels: the damaging manifestations range from encouraging a sedentary lifestyle, to robbing children of healthy interactive relationships, to barricading their willingness and interest in constructive responsibilities such as chores or homework.[83]

Then, later:

Worse than this, between the ages of two and six years old, the brain finishes most of its physical development, reaching 90% of its adult capacity.[84] During this time, and particularly between the ages of four and five, a process called synaptic pruning takes place: "neurons that are seldom stimulated lose their connective fibers, and the number of synapses gradually declines."[85] What takes place during this process is the brain's selection of which neural connectors to fine-tune, and which to slowly "phaseout." In a nutshell, neural connections within the brain which are not being stimulated are at risk of atrophy.[86]

As if this isn't bad enough, Anderson goes on to explain that dopamine is released during some interaction with technology, a sensation that drives such new epidemics as video-gaming addiction, which is proving to be accompanied by urges for screen time comparable to that of drug cravings.[87] When children are allowed to become addicted to media, and are denied, they can experience mood swings, depression, and other behaviors not unlike those of people who are addicted to chemical substances. (This is due to the decline in dopamine as a result of screen deprivation.)

Hours spent interacting with media feeds isolation and loneliness (a great disadvantage to good health). Additionally, a child's capacity to utilize and hone all five senses during the developmental phases is disabled, which can inhibit him or her in countless psychological *and* physical ways throughout his or her lifetime. This is made worse when we consider that the secluded, still-developing child will—thanks to media—be "exposed to as many as twenty acts of violence every hour, while other statistics reveal that the average child in America will witness up to twelve thousand acts of violence per year through this activity."[88] What this means is that children who overindulge in digital interaction experience diminished intellectual development, illusions about the real world (via social media), remain sedentary, miss vital physical developmental cues, and potentially lose out on segments of their ability to emotionally connect with others—all while witnessing repetitive violence.

These authors both challenge and beg you to examine the technological balance (or imbalance) within your home and make any corrections you can to ensure the psychological and physical health of everyone in your household.

Isolation v. Community

Two of the biggest inhibitors to good health are loneliness and isolation. While these may sound like two words for the same thing, they're not. Loneliness springs from limited interaction with others, while isolation is the feeling of being disconnected from others. Some people can be in a room filled with people and still feel isolated, while others who spend a considerable amount of time by themselves may not necessarily feel lonely. And, while these might seem like strictly social issues, they actually have a large capability to influence our health in physical ways. Medical research regarding the elderly has recently established significant links between these two factors and various psychological and physical health conditions such as "high blood pressure, heart disease, obesity, a weakened immune system, anxiety, depression, cognitive decline, Alzheimer's disease, and even death."[89] On the other hand, those who engage in fulfilling acts with others in a setting of family, social support, or community find that such interaction improves positive thought patterns, reinforces healthy cognitive processes, and even promotes longer life.[90] Doctors John and Stephanie Cacioppo, in their studies on loneliness and isolation and the impact on health, social integration, and general lifespan, concluded that "loneliness automatically triggers a set of related behavioral and biological processes that contribute to the association between loneliness and premature death in people of all ages."[91]

It may seem obvious that one of the ways loneliness and isolation affect a person is because both can allow thoughts to migrate toward negativity. But there's more to it than this. According to Dr. Steve Cole of the University of California's Social Genomics Core Laboratory, the mistrust experienced by a person who feels this way will trigger a defense response within his or her biological makeup. For example, negative feelings may cause the body's defense mechanism to trigger inflammation, which is both the body's response to injury and at times can promote the healing of injury. But long-term inflammation also contributes to chronic illness. Dr. Cole states that in this and other ways, loneliness is "a fertilizer for other diseases."[92] Elaborating on this link between loneliness/isolation and other diseases, he adds that a compromised immune system leaves an individual vulnerable to other viruses and infectious diseases.[93]

Some statements asserted by prominent experts regarding the link between loneliness/isolation and mental/physical health are stunning. For example, Dr. Julianne Holt-Lunstad, a professor of psychology and neuroscience, notes that "lack of social connection heightens health risks as much as smoking 15 cigarettes a day or having alcohol use disorder… [and that] loneliness and social isolation are twice as harmful to physical and mental health as obesity."[94] Lunstad also states that interpersonal connection is a necessity "crucial to...well-being and survival."[95]

Yes, you read that right. Let's give that a minute to sink in. Loneliness and isolation are *twice* as harmful to your health as obesity. Furthermore, the heightened health risk is comparable to smoking fifteen cigarettes a day or regularly abusing alcohol!

How can this be?

In the beginning, we see that God created man, and said, "It is not good that the man should be alone; I will make him...[a companion]" (Genesis 2:19). When God looked upon the man and woman he had made in His own image (Genesis 1:27), He told them to be fruitful, multiply, and replenish the earth. Why? Because God wired mankind for *community*. No one should be alone. This doesn't necessarily mean that every person *should* get married, nor does it suggest that a person can't live alone. Some people are very happy having their own space or remaining single. But it *does* mean that we all have the fundamental need to be plugged into some sort of community. Many who are lonely or isolated don't even realize that *this* is the cause of their suffering. The symptoms surround us daily; Look at how oversexualized our society is. This is a byproduct of the widespread lack of intimacy many people are suffer. Perhaps you've noticed how many people are sending samples of their DNA to companies promising to link them to ancestral connections. This, for many, is a way to make up for a lack of family association. Social media promises friendships, but often becomes the basis of a cruel, unobtainable game of comparison. The list of ways loneliness and isolation manifest in our time and place goes on and on. The commonality among all the symptoms is this: They are offshoots of a lack of community.

We can't stress enough how vital it is for your holistic well-being— your spiritual, psychological, and physical health—that you find a community outlet and become part of it. Perhaps it is church, a mentoring program, or a volunteer position at a local school, food drive, or library. Or, you might find connection with others via activities that don't necessarily involve volunteerism, such as taking a dance class or joining a book club. The possibilities are all around.

This advice may seem to run counter to our earlier encouragement to consider cutting some activities from your schedule. The difference is this: Work that is obligatory, dreaded, or for pay often doesn't yield the positive friendship and interpersonal rewards as community involvement. *Sometimes we must set aside good things to make room for better things.* That doesn't mean that what we eliminate isn't valuable, but rather, there are some things that cannot be traded. Once you have created space in your life by editing out some of the activities that drain you, you'll probably find it intriguing to pursue your interests and surround yourself with others who enjoy similar things.

For many (even those who suffer from loneliness/isolation), the idea of making new friends is completely intimidating. For one thing, busy schedules make maintaining a friendship seem impossible (hence the notion of creating space). For others, trusting is hard. But good friendships are both necessary and rewarding. There is a time in everyone's life when God will send us a friend to enhance our joy. I (Daniel) believe an intervening friend comes into our lives at the right time when we are receptive, an individual whose very presence has life-changing value. This exchange is mutual, although sometimes it may seem like one is helping the other more, depending on the season. Often, one friend's knowledge or influence will be just what the other needs that moment. Later, the two may (and probably should) exchange roles. For me (Daniel), that person was a girlfriend years ago who had good information that I needed, and who believed in me. For Joe, Mark Taylor and Joshua Vance offered good knowledge alongside companionship that he considers life-changing. When we begin to foster bonds such as these, we have a greater understanding of our ultimate Friend who sticks closer than a brother: Jesus (Proverbs 18:24).

Scientific Proof

Telomeres

Science proves that our choices affect our long-term health and can even lengthen our lives. This evidence is found in what science calls telomeres. Telomeres are a vital part of our cells, located at the end of each strand of DNA, that protect and encase the chromosomes within. The condition of telomeres varies from person to person, depending on our health, and directly correlate with the aging and degenerative processes. Regardless of our chronological age, they offer an estimation of our biological age. As we become ill, expose the body to compromising materials or substances, or even as a byproduct of stress, telomeres gradually wear down. As a result, our lifestyles impact the length of these gene-protecting agents, meaning death moves closer on our timeline. In other words, the shorter the telomere, the closer we are to the date of death. However, there is good news. Studies have shown that diminishing of these sleeve-like DNA caps can be either dramatically slowed, halted, or *even reversed* (dramatic reversal is rarer and depends on the situation). Because they are affected by lifestyle, stress level, diet, activity, individual happiness, sleep regimen, and more, we can begin to reclaim telomere length by making positive changes in our lives.

Understand that, when we discuss telomeres and the issue of decisions, we're looking at ways to change your well-being that don't require any special status or financial investment, gym memberships, or specialized medical therapy. You may be surprised to learn that 80 percent of the health of these life-determining gene-sleeves can be changed for the better by the *everyday choices that we make.*

Have you ever parted ways with a friend, then reunited several years later to see that they somehow looked younger than in previous years? (We touched on this earlier, in our discussion about obesity). Surely, upon inquiring, you learn that the friend made some life changes that increased his or her happiness or relieved stress. We've all known people who have been in an abusive relationship, a high-tension or demanding job, or otherwise had a life filled with unhealthy indulgences, and we've seen the evidence show on their body and in their countenance. Seeing such people make adaptations to their lives often slows or reverses the aging process.

Another liberating factor when considering telomeres is that we know we aren't powerless. While we don't always have a choice in whether we suffer, we can take solace in the fact that we determine whether our suffering will continue to escalate unchecked. This is no anomaly before God. He has placed control of many physical and psychological issues in our very own hands.

Epigenetic Expressions

Epigenome is another term you may have heard related to health issues. It refers to a construct of proteins and body chemicals that can attach to DNA and literally activate or deactivate genes. Research has shown that "lifestyle…[such as] nutrition, behavior, stress, physical activity, working habits, smoking and alcohol consumption…[and] environmental… factors may influence epigenetic mechanisms."[96] In short, the decisions we make and the way we live can turn on certain parts of our genetic makeup while subverting others completely. The indication is that, even if we fear the worst for our genetic alignment, we can alter by making choices that cause it to turn on positive, immune-supporting genes, while suppressing those that cause excessive inflammation, chemical or hormone imbalance, or leave us vulnerable to illness. This literally gives us the cognitive power to influence the expression or depression of our own gene extension.

Mitochondrial Biogenesis

Another term you'll hear throughout this book is "mitochondria." These are sack-type structures in cells that convert materials to energy, process fat, and initiate cell regeneration. The inner lining of the mitochondria has many "folds," for lack of a better word, and within these folds dwell proteins that help create energy through a complicated chemical exchange process called the Krebs, or citric acid, cycle.[97] One cell could have hundreds or even thousands of mitochondria within, and these fascinating elements work with seeming autonomy within our bodies to keep us healthy. They can destroy neighboring damaged mitochondrial cells, even by functioning independently or networking together. They contribute to muscular, neurological, cognitive, hormonal, and metabolic stability and health, and their dysfunction can compromise well-being or even cause fatality.

As we age, our mitochondrial functions deteriorate. The more rapidly this drop occurs, the more quickly we age. This contributes to why some folks may appear physically older or younger than their age: mitochondrial care, function, and activity largely dictates our youthfulness and well-being throughout adult life. Similarly, as these microorganisms age, they often experience a decline in energy production, malfunction, or even mutate, lending vulnerability to the onset of disorder or disease. Preserving the health and stability of our mitochondrial genes ensures the same for our overall health.

However, studies have shown that in the early processes of aging, the communication between mitochondria and the host cell is disturbed as a result of chemical degradation over time. To put it into everyday language, the cell sends inadequate signals to the mitochondria requesting energy, which results in the mitochondrial output being less than requested.[98] This causes a rundown state to perpetuate within cells, opening the door to aging and illness. But, if we can maintain our mitochondrial well-being and open lines of communication between these entities and their hosts at an early enough stage, we can potentially delay or even reverse the aging process.[99] Many researchers are looking into ways of replenishing cell chemicals that would bolster this communication, but mitochondria respond to the conditions of our daily lives. If we practice healthy living, we preserve the vitality of these important microorganisms, and vice versa.

Our bodies are capable of initiating a process called mitochondrial biogenesis, which refers to shedding damaged or unhealthy mitochondria and regenerating new ones. This is induced by placing just enough stress on the system that it triggers what is known as mitohormesis, the body's response to an element that, in small doses, is beneficial, but in larger quantities can be detrimental. Exercise is a prime example of this. When the mitohormesis response has initiated, the body produces a protein called PGC-1 alpha, which then deploys mitochondrial biogenesis.[100] The body rejuvenates cells, removes dead or dying cellular tissue, and refurbishes it with a new, healthy supply. This prevents illness and keeps the quality of life high by helping us feel vibrant, youthful, energetic, healthy, and emotionally balanced. Other ways of inducing mitochondrial biogenesis—such as cold shock, heat shock, fasting, and ketones—will be discussed at more length throughout the book.

The Answers Simplify

Interesting to note in searching for the keys to good health is that the more we seek answers, the simpler they become. The large, life-changing revelations that we often look for are usually so small that they can only be seen with a microscope. So many people are looking to heal organs such as the liver, lungs, heart, pancreas, and so on, but all too often we overlook the very building blocks those organs are made *from*. When we take interest in healing our bodies on a cellular level, we find ourselves, again, seeing redundantly basic and yet often overlooked themes: sleep, diet, and exercise. It is blissfully liberating that such guileless answers are at the center of our search. Essentially, we can obtain *much* of the relief we seek via our own choices. By focusing on fostering healthy cells, we receive the benefit of having vigorous bodies. If the cells that make up our organs are in good shape, then these tissues are inclined to follow suit.

Meditation and Prayer

There is an increasing interest in the scientific and medical fields regarding the power of prayer and meditation. In fact, a study released by the University of Rochester stated that more than 85 percent of people facing serious illness pray. Some experts assert that prayer and meditation are powerful tools, while others scoff, placing placebo-type labels on these activities. (Ironically, the very fact that a placebo has an effect is, in itself, validation of the point.) However, as we've discussed, just as the defense response triggered by the body causes inflammation, compromised immunity, and imbalance of body chemicals and hormones, prayer and meditation have been discovered to trigger an *opposing* response. This is known as "the relaxation response...[wherein] the body's metabolism decreases, the heart rate slows, blood pressure goes down, and... [breathing] becomes calmer and more regular."[101] Genes that would dispatch inflammation throughout the body are disabled, and brainwaves that occur during the relaxation response are correlated with feelings of empowerment, tranquility, and control. Considering that more than half of the visits to American doctors' offices are for treatment of illnesses to which stress, depression, and anxiety greatly contribute, it becomes clear that "the relaxation response" can be seen as a type of preventative medicine for chronic illness.

University of Pennsylvania's Dr. Andrew Newberg conducted a study on prayer and meditation and found that those who pray/meditate experience increased levels of dopamine, the hormone and neurotransmitter associated with happiness and a sense of well-being. Furthermore, the National Institute of Health funded a study that revealed that people who pray are "40 percent less likely to have high blood pressure"[102] than those who do not, which contributes to better relaxation, stress management, and quality and quantity of sleep. Dartmouth Medical researchers indicate that patients who persistently hold spiritual values are "three times more likely to recover" than those who don't have such values.[103] The list of studies linking prayer and meditation to wellness and healing abound, and, whether or not a person believes in God, these revelations support an argument for such practices.

Prayer sets the mind on the positive and fills it with hope. Faith grows when we pray, and stress is relieved when we realize we're not alone, and that we have a higher force to lean on and ask for help. Likewise, prayer relaxes the body, remedies inner turmoil that contributes to illness, and gives us better control over our thought patterns. The benefits are spiritual, mental, *and* physical.

The subjects we've discussed in this chapter are the primary steps to creating a new life for yourself and your loved ones. You can implement them while you begin to learn more about how your body interacts with nature in the upcoming pages. We prayerfully hope you'll start to make these changes and find healing in Jesus' Name.

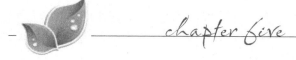

chapter five

Circadian Rhythm

To every thing there is a season, and a time to
every purpose under the heaven.
~ECCLESIASTES 3:1

Many refer to the body as having some type of "clock." When certain parts of the country change to Daylight Savings Time or when we cross time zones in our travels, for example, we complain that it throws off our "internal clock." When we discuss life chapters such as those defined by childbearing or retirement, we refer to a "biological clock." A newborn infant who cries for feeding at 3 a.m. is a prime example of one whose timing hasn't yet been conditioned to life outside the womb. When we refer to our bodies having some sort of internal timing mechanism, we're closer to accuracy than even we realize, yet many don't recognize the name of the most important internal clock that we have: circadian rhythm. Further, to say that the body has a built-in timekeeper may give the impression that this mechanism merely regulates when we wake up, become hungry, and go back to sleep. But, it does so much more; it controls the entire functionality of our physical makeup. And, it embodies one simple truth that many of us don't realize: The timing of our bodily systems is often just as important—if not more so—as what we actually *do* with our bodies. While the circadian rhythm is often overlooked or taken for granted by people going about their daily lives, there are vast ways it is vital to our overall health.

What Is Circadian Rhythm?

The word "circadian" is generated from the roots *circa* ("around") and *dian* (or *diam,* "day").[104] So the concept refers to a cycle in which our body is meant to work "around the day." This is an internal clock that is active for the entire twenty-four-hour period. For the human body, the clock is divided into three segments wherein the activity is geared toward a specific theme: sleep, nutrition, and activity. Almost every gene, hormone, and biochemical mechanism turns on and off at different times of the day. These genes govern nearly every aspect of our lives, like inflammation, energy, sleep, memory, and healing, just to name a few. All aspects of our DNA are woven into this internal timekeeper, which is synchronized through a paired group of neurons in the hypothalamus. This master clock in the brain is called the suprachiasmatic nucleus (SCN), a tiny cerebral feature that is made up of a whopping twenty-thousand brain cells, and which is set to respond to light signals relayed via the protein melanopsin, which is located within the retina of the eye.[105] The SCN is located above the optic nerves that cross at the center of the brain. It keeps tabs on the light signals brought in through the eyes and discerns which type of light it is seeing. Depending on the type of light it's picking up on, it sends cues throughout the body regulating appetite, motivation for activity, hormone generation and secretion, body temperature, and even moods. Surprisingly, even blind people are able to pick up enough light sensation to keep the SCN informed.

The circadian cycle is an innate feature that has evolved across the centuries to preserve our ability to hunt, gather, work, and remain vigilant during the waking hours of the day. In a (hypothetical) world in which there is nothing to interrupt it, here's a basic idea of how circadian rhythm works:

———

In the morning, sunlight (often referred to as "blue light") comes peering through the windows, filtering through the melanopsin light sensors in the retina. The eyes process these rays toward the SCN, which alerts you to the fact that a new day has begun. The pineal gland then dispatches hormones such as cortisol to cause you to rise. The pancreas is on standby, ready to dispatch the insulin necessary to metabolize breakfast. At around 9 a.m., testosterone and attentiveness should reach their peak, providing you the strength and energy you need to face the work day ahead. Shortly thereafter, your physical coordination escalates and cardiovascular strength increases. (These are adaptations that have formed over years of mankind's need for the great manual labor known by our ancestors.) During the first half of the day, your body is in the segment of the cycle that leans toward nutrition. During these hours, insulin levels are healthiest and food is processed best. This is when the system is most efficient about pulling nutrients out of the food that's been ingested. Similarly, bowel movements often happen in the first half of day, the body having conducted its own detox-and-purge process during the night. By about noon, your mental function is at its height, and after this stimulating period of time, your physical body becomes its sharpest in early- to mid-afternoon. By evening, your blood pressure reaches its high point, as the body begins to prepare for its nightly detox regime, which takes place during sleep. In response to this heightened blood pressure, your body temperature spikes at around 7 p.m. As your activity diminishes and blue light decreases and eventually disappears, the body eliminates chemicals that foster alertness. Melatonin kicks in at around 9 p.m., causing you to become sleepy. By about 10 p.m., sleep sets in, and by 2 a.m., you should be experiencing the deepest sleep of the night. During this time, your brain is processing, storing, and filing memories of events that took place during the day. The brain is likewise conducting a mass detox process, ridding your systems of toxins you we were exposed to over the day. In like manner, it is finishing the absorption process of nutrients you took in while you were awake, and is even producing such vital chemicals as melatonin, hormones, and human growth hormone, a vital element in the growth of children and injury healing in adults.

This continues until approximately 4 a.m., when your body begins to undergo the physical changes that prepare you for waking up, despite your obliviousness to this transition. Melatonin production decreases, you temperature and blood pressure increase, and breathing speeds up slightly. Your eyes open, you wake up, and the circadian rhythm repeats.

———

As stated previously, this cycle has evolved throughout the history of mankind, adapting to environmental demands. Along these lines, it's interesting that while everyone's circadian routine is approximately twenty-four hours long, the precise timing can vary slightly among individuals. For example, in the aforementioned example, 10 p.m. is the time sleep sets in. However, some people move in slightly earlier or later rotations. The result is the variance that we would use when referring to people as "morning larks" or "night owls." Why such a discrepancy? Matthew Walker explains that our ancestors were wired to:

...co-sleep as families or even whole tribes...the benefits of such variation in sleep/wake timing preferences can be understood. The night owls...[would fall asleep] between one or two a.m.... the morning larks...would have retired at 9 p.m. and woken at 5 a.m. Consequently, the group as a whole is only collectively vulnerable...for just four hours rather than eight hours.[106]

The scenario described earlier, to someone juggling many responsibilities, may seem like a pipe dream. In this day and age, such a schedule seems hardly obtainable considering our busy lifestyles. Yet, our cycles define how our bodies were meant to thrive. Have you ever wondered why people in our grandparents' generation, many of them farmers, managed to stay so healthy into such late ages? If we examine their diets, we find a paradox. Their food was organic/farm raised (a positive contribution to their health!) but what they ate was often filled with fats and carbs—a diet doctors would steer today's patients *away* from. Foods such as eggs, bread, gravy, and bacon were eaten regularly, while fresh fruits and vegetables may have only been available seasonally. However, due to the lack of television, the Internet, and other distractions, they often spent evenings in decreased activity, and when it was dark outside, the great majority went to sleep. When we scrutinize their lifestyles, we find that they lived in accordance with the ideal daily cycle. Each of the three themes of the circadian were honored: sleep (regulated by the sun's rising and setting); nutrition (through the farming of safe and wholesome food); and activity (through manual labor and the habit of finding entertainment through activity and healthy social settings).

For some, it may seem that if we work against our own cycle long enough, it will eventually change. After all, those who fly to different regions of the world experience jet lag, but they soon recover. However, travel involves the fact that, in the new region, *sunlight* is operating on a different timeline—so, after a day or two, the body adapts. Working in a time zone where the body must operate against the sun has direr consequences. University of California in Berkeley's professor of neuroscience, Dr. Matthew Walker, states:

> Wakefulness and sleep are therefore under the control of the circadian rhythm, and not the other way around...[it] will march up and down every twenty-four hours irrespective of whether you have slept or not.[107]

This is particularly true for shift workers who must remain awake during nocturnal hours when their cycle wishes for sleep.

These folks are regularly pushing against their body's preferred cycle, and the manifestation of this physical taxation can have measurable disadvantages. A study in *Occupational and Environmental Medicine* found that employees who held such shifts "had lower scores on tests of memory, processing speed and overall brain power…[and experienced] cognitive deficits so steep that the study authors equated them to 6.5 years of age related decline."[108]

Just like shift workers, the body's organs and glands—such as the liver and the thyroid—do different jobs at different times of the day. In a production plant, an exact order of operations has to happen to produce a final product: If anyone is unable to properly carry out his or her responsibilities, the result is likely to be a defective product. For us, this means that timing is everything. For example, eating a bagel in the morning means that the liver has adequate time and prepared support to efficiently take in the calories, which will generally be burned throughout the day instead of becoming stored fat. However, eating the same bagel in the evening will result in the bagel being converted to stored fat. As we'll explain a little later, *what* we eat isn't all that matters where diet is concerned; it is also *when* we're eating that's significant.

Light

Limiting our exposure to technology can add quality to our lives. While the sun is the greatest source of blue light, electronic screens produce a similar light in diminished capacity—not enough to supplement the lack of natural daylight—but adequate amounts to throw the body into wakefulness during the evening hours when the body should be preparing for sleep. You may think, "I can wind down with television just fine. I still get to sleep without trouble," but unfortunately you may not be aware of the chemical alterations that your body *should have* gone through but didn't, and thus aren't privy to the declined quality of your sleep. Those who watch excessive television in the evening, stare at a computer too many hours late into the day, or even enjoy too much phone time during this segment of the cycle stunt melatonin development and harm their health by means of sleep deprivation.

On the other hand, lack of sunlight can tell the brain's mechanism to falsely believe that it is dark outside, resulting in the generating of melatonin at sporadic times during the day. Often, our workplaces have limited natural light, which, coupled with sitting in a chair at a desk for too long, can trigger sleepiness. This often contributes to the need for additional coffee—a solution that, incidentally, doesn't address the actual problem. The *real* issue in such a case is not the lack of caffeine, but is rather a deficiency of *sunlight*.

All this talk of sunlight may draw us to believe that circadian rhythm is a response system to our external world rather than a force from within. It would be simple to buy into the notion that when the sun comes up, we wake, and when it goes down, we sleep—just like clockwork. However, studies that began in the 1950s have shown that this timekeeper remains true, guiding human beings along a cycle roughly twenty-four hours and fifteen minutes in duration, even when we're completely locked away from the influence of the sun, moon, and other cosmic markers of time. Further, although circadian rhythm is largely cued by blue light, other triggers influence (even *throw off*) its timing as well, including food intake, exercise, and blue light exposure at the wrong times of day. (We will talk about this more a little later.)

In the 1950s, a volunteer ventured far into a cave in the Andes mountains carrying only the simplest provisions: enough food to survive on for several weeks, some candles, and reading material. A rudimentary telephone was designed that could only call out to log the time to a volunteer. Each time the hiker felt sleep setting in, he'd report via telephone, and would do the same as he woke up. The experiment showed that his internal clock operated with near-perfect precision, with one exception: He woke up slightly later each day, and retired in the same fashion. In total, his cycle showed a pattern of being twenty-four hours and fifteen minutes long, but despite his clock being slightly longer than twenty-four hours, his rhythm was consistent for the duration of his cave-dwelling time. What was gleaned from these findings was that although adequate blue light or sunlight can *trigger* or sometimes even *reset* this internal timekeeper, it exists within our innate mechanisms, independent of our environment, and hardwired into our brains as a separate entity from the outside world. This proves that while our systems are able to adapt, we must follow the cycle for which we're designed.

Drumming Against the Rhythm

When circadian rhythm is disrupted, negative changes can begin to take place in as little as a few days. After this short time, our genes begin receiving corrupt signals, resulting in compromised immunity that allows the onset of infections and other diseases, insomnia and cognitive/psychological malfunctions, migraines, diabetes, obesity, and even serious illness such as cardiovascular disease and/or cancer.

Throughout this chapter, you may see the term "shift worker," so it is best to describe it before moving on: Salk Institute professor and founding executive member at the University of California in San Diego's Center for Circadian Biology, Satchin Panda, a leading researcher into the science surrounding the circadian rhythm, defines it as someone who is awake more than three hours per night, more than fifty nights per year, between the hours of 10 p.m. and 5 a.m.[109] As we learn more about this vital, yet all-too-often disregarded mechanism, the more correlations surface between its disruption and serious physical and psychological health issues. In fact, night-shift work has become known to be a potential health hazard because of its ability to disrupt the circadian rhythm. Some experts now believe that heart disease is related to circadian rhythm. The link between interruption of the circadian rhythm and cancer has become so evident in studies of shift workers that "in 2007, the World Health Organization's International Agency for Research on Cancer classified shift work as a potential carcinogen."[110]

Timing Food Intake

We mentioned previously that elements other than light can cue the circadian rhythm. Food intake is one of the largest factors negatively impacting our internal timekeepers, and its abuse does more damage than we realize. As previously said, *when* we eat matters as much as *what we eat*.

In 2009, an experiment was conducted wherein nocturnal mice were deprived of food during their normal eating hours (which would have been during the night), and instead were only fed during the day. Soon, it was revealed that "almost every liver gene that turns on and off within 24 hours completely tracked the food and ignored the timing of light exposure."[111] This means that while blue light is the most obvious trigger for the internal clock, food is capable of completely taking its place, causing "food to reset the liver clock, not the brain."[112] The body is able to take opposing cues from differing sources and adapt varying organs to function with independent timing. In other words, light tells our brains what segment of the cycle we're are in, but food intake, when ill-timed (pun intended), communicates a *different* cycle to our organs, causing the system to fight against itself.

Because the cycle is inclined toward nutrition for the first segment of the day, our bodies enter physiological stages during the morning hours that set us up for optimal digestion and organ function. For example, morning light causes the brain and gut to communicate hunger signals to one another, priming the pancreas for insulin secretion. The muscles, which are preparing for manual labor, begin searching for incoming nutrition, and the body enters a type of "fat-storage" mode. (Don't let this phrase intimidate you and don't decline eating in the morning for fear of ruining your diet. The truth is, this is an optimal setting.) The science can seem complicated, but in a nutshell: When you eat, the body goes into a mode for storing fat, which it plans to subsequently turn into energy to carry you throughout the day. When you're through eating and the body realizes no more food is coming, it switches into a "fat-burning" mode, wherein food just taken in is now *used* as energy. This conversion takes approximately two hours. Thus, nutrition taken in during the early portion of the day is temporarily stored as fat the body burns throughout the day. (Recall that the circadian rhythm has evolved over the centuries, and previous generations would have eaten breakfast and then done vast amounts of manual labor for the waking, daylight hours). As you go about your day, these calories are burned by activity, until sometime around midday, you get hungry again. The process of fat-storage/fat-burning repeats for the early and middle parts of the day, because these calories are stored in anticipation of the prime physical activity the body foresees for the upcoming afternoon.

After about eight to ten hours of food intake over the course of the day, the organs that process this influx begin to wind down and prepare for sleep. While the digestion process during the first part of the day can typically be completed within a couple of hours, after this time window, it takes significantly longer, because the gut and other digestive organs need rest. The consequence at this point is that the system, which "cannot make and break up body fat at the same time,"[113] is forced to store virtually all food intake as fat cells. As mentioned, food taken in and stored as fat begins to be burned after a couple hours, then the body switches from the fat storage setting to the burning setting. However, because the body is entering the sleep state and attempting to begin nightly detox processes, the fat-burning stage doesn't engage until morning, when it is further confused by incoming nutrients and its self-determined position to instead switch into the storage mode. Thus, calories consumed at night become true manifestation of the old adage: "a moment on the lips, a lifetime on the hips." Damage is caused to organs that must behave erratically just to find and maintain their place in a cycle that is being continually jarred by mixed signals.

This is why late-night snacking is devastating to our bodies. Since the pancreas, stomach, liver, and even muscles by this point are entering the pre-sleep mode while the body allows the blood pressure and temperature to spike as it begins to focus on an upcoming night of detox, these mixed signals confuse the organs. They were preparing for sleep, but now have to shift focus from the necessary routine activities to dealing with a sudden influx of unexpected (and uninvited) food. It throws their clock backward by several hours, launching them into a mode they would have been prepared for many hours earlier, but are not prepared for now. The timing is simply off. Digestive juices are not secreted, and the liver, which was preparing itself for the night's detox procedures, is occupied with other tasks. This launches the body into a type of emergency state to handle this unanticipated development. Other organs receive the message that intake is occurring, and, misunderstanding what hour of the day it is, they either speed up or slow way down in an attempt to re-sync themselves to the appropriate time. (Have you ever had a day that left you exhausted and hungry, but after you ate, you were unable to sleep? Bingo.) As all of these cogs within the wheel of the internal pacekeeper panic and autonomously attempt to assess and rectify their timing, the overall system is thrown out of whack. Additionally, because the body takes about two hours to switch from the "fat-storage" to "fat-burning" settings, sporadic eating keeps the body suspended in "fat-storage" mode for lack of opportunity to transition, causing everything we eat to be stored as fat. This impedes the ability of the pancreas to process and balance sugar and insulin levels, which leads to diabetes.[114]

And we do this to ourselves every single night, don't we?

Intermittent Fasting

The catastrophic impact of eating around the clock—as so many of us do—is cause for alarm, but there may be comfort for the reader in knowing that this problem has a very simple solution: intermittent fasting. Now, before you're swept into the fear of the unknown, or the simpler but real terror of having to go hungry, hear us out. We've already hinted at intermittent fasting, but we'll elaborate here. While some extremists may boast of their ability to fast for days on end, adding this practice to your everyday life can take on a much easier application. And, while some small sacrifice is still involved, the health benefits are literally immeasurable.

As a society, our eating habits have morphed over the decades. Whereas we used to eat three regular meals a day, we've added to this traditional eating style the model of snacking between every meal. In addition, the continual invasion of technology into our lives has resulted in a majority of people staying up much later in the evening hours than previous generations. These late-night indulgences are often accompanied with more munching. The result of this is that, by and large, we eat almost around the clock, and this is a workload our digestive organs were never designed for. As already explained, continual intake keeps a person's body in the "fat storage" mode, but in addition, it overworks the gut, liver, and pancreas, which causes them to eventually wear out and even malfunction prematurely. (Imagine owning a car, but instead of turning it off when it's parked, you always leave the vehicle idling, allowing no rest period. Eating around the clock places extra "miles" on vital tissues for no important purpose, and bring no fruitful yield in return.) Further, as stated, this nonstop influx greatly contributes to diabetes, impedes weight loss, and even impacts sleep. However, intermittent fasting can help reverse many of these cycles and set the body's systems back into harmony. When we're fasting, we spend more hours at a time in an uninterrupted, fat-burning state. Insulin levels decrease, causing the body to turn to stored fat for energy, which actually speeds up the ability to lose weight while giving such organs as the gut, liver, and pancreas time to rejuvenate between jobs, restoring efficacy to the entire metabolic function. Human growth hormone increases, which causes lean muscle to form, in turn promoting healthy caloric expulsion. Beyond this, the physiological changes that take place during a fast improve cognitive function and help reduce chances of such illness as cancer, blood pressure issues, and even ailments such as Alzheimer's and Parkinson's diseases.[115]

Having already mentioned mitochondrial biogenesis, we won't dwell on the subject here other than to recall the fact that intermittent fasting is one of the ways to initiate this cellular healing process.

The circadian clock and the timing of food intake directly impact the effectiveness of our metabolism and immune system and affects our inclination toward chronic illness, our cognitive function, and even our neurological health. As mentioned in the previous chapter, what we choose to engage in for the sake of our health can actually alter the condition of our cells and even change our genome. To learn more about this phenomenon, researchers came together from the University of California, the Baylor College of Medicine in Houston, Texas, and the Telethon Institute of Genetics and Medicine in Naples, Italy, to study the impact of feeding-pattern alteration on the genetic expression of mice. They found that intermittent fasting caused gene expression to incline toward prevention of aging, illness, and disease. The study revealed that "the reorganization of gene regulation by fasting could prime the genome to…anticipate upcoming food intake and thereby drive a new rhythmic cycle of gene expression… Therefore, optimal [intermittent] fasting…[could] positively affect cellular functions and…[benefit] health and…[prevent] aging-associated diseases."[116] (We'll discuss how this is scientifically possible in the upcoming pages.)

Furthermore, the *New England Journal of Medicine* released an article in 2019, written by doctors Raphael de Cabo and Mark P. Patterson, which looked into the matter as well. The piece asserted that intermittent fasting initiates "adaptive cellular responses that are integrated between and within organs in a manner that improves glucose regulation, increases stress resistance, and suppresses inflammation."[117] Further, they stated that "preclinical studies show the robust disease-modifying efficacy... on a wide range of chronic disorders, including obesity, diabetes, cardiovascular disease, cancers, and neurodegenerative brain diseases."[118] Other benefits were included in the report as well. Cellular fortitude in healthy cells was reinforced, creating better resistance to diseases such as cancer. Cognitive function saw improvements as it pertains to spatial, associative, and working memory, illustrating that fasting can be beneficial even to those who don't believe they are struggling with chronic illness. Harmony between organs' functions was restored, causing overall systemic efficacy to improve.[119]

Autophagy

At this point, you may be wondering how it is possible that so many benefits can come from taking in minimal nutrients. The notion seems counterintuitive; after all, haven't we always believed that eating nutritious food will arm our bodies to fight illness? How is it, then, that nutrient deprivation can drive our bodies toward myriad healthy, rejuvenating processes?

When we don't eat for a period of time, the lack of food initiates a process called autophagy. The word, literally meaning "self-eating,"[120] describes the survival mechanism by which the body begins to forage within itself for dead cells that it can consume as an alternative to incoming nutrition. This is the physiological response to the realization that food has been restricted. The system shifts into a type of survival mode, increasing efficiency by scavenging throughout its own system in search for material that can be eaten, reabsorbed, and recreated into new energy.[121] The best part of this process is that as it seeks out old or damaged cells and recycles them, the body likewise releases newer, healthier cells to replace them. Because this response is activated by self-scavenging, it prioritizes the weakest, most damaged, or degenerate cells.

A similar way to look at this process is if you were to suddenly be required to downsize your wardrobe, and were told that there is no guarantee of when new clothing will be available. You would operate with the realization that you must make careful choices as to what to keep or discard, understanding that this new, smaller wardrobe may have to last a while. Clothing that is worn out, torn, faded, threadbare, or otherwise close to its expiration will likely be thrown out first, while you'll probably hold on to newer or better items. After your effort, you would have fewer items of clothing, but you would also have a wardrobe that is, overall, in better condition. In the same way, autophagy looks discriminately through the system for cells that are more useful to the body when burned as fuel than left as living cells, thus prioritizing those that are degenerate or unhealthy to be consumed. After a length of time in this process, you will have fewer degenerate and nutrient-leeching cells; you will have lost weight; and you will find that scrutiny of the remaining cells shows them to be in generally better condition.

Autophagy relieves inflammation, restores the immune system, contributes to insulin balance, and prevents and fights chronic illness. Not only does this process have beneficial detox properties, but this continual rejuvenation of cellular health alters gene expression, restoring health and delaying or even reversing the aging process.

Before a Fast

When the body is given food, its sense of threat is diminished; thus, all cells are nourished—even those that aren't healthy. At the cellular level, communication pathways called mTORs (mammalian target of rapamycin), send signals regarding insulin and incoming nutrients.[122] In a fed state, these have proteins that keep the division and growth (reproduction) of these cells occurring regularly. (This process is the opposite of autophagy, mentioned previously, which is the recycling of dead or degenerate cells.) When mTOR pathways are overstimulated for long periods, they show a correlation to cancer cell development.[123] When this part of the cellular makeup is in production mode (well-fed state), they have the power to disable the parts of the genome that efficiently facilitate fat metabolism, healing and reparation, inflammation, and even stress management.[124] However, during a fast, they have the potential to be reversed: the well-fed status of mTORs is switched to the nutrient-deprived state, while genes yielding benefits just mentioned are switched back on, a reversal process that is partially facilitated by ketones (agents created by the liver to balance insulin when food intake is diminished for a period; more on this later). This reversal is instigated by the AMPK (activated protein kinase) pathways—signaling units that alert the activation of self-preservation extremes. Via this transfer of orders on a cellular level, the body engages its response to threat: self-preserving mechanisms are triggered that increase the body's efficacy with existing nutrients; foster an alternate, self-made form of insulin (ketones); and release resources designed to help the system operate with diminished sensations of stress despite increasingly worrying circumstances (lack of incoming nutrients). As AMPK orders are followed throughout the physiology, mTOR's growth, division, and reproduction orders are ceased in favor of autophagy, mitochondrial biogenesis, antioxidant processes, cell repair and rejuvenation, fat breakdown, and use of general resources.[125]

What Happens During a Fast

When you've been fasting for twelve hours, your body enters a stage called ketosis.[126] During this time, stored fat begins to be tapped by the liver in order to produce ketones, an alternative to glucose. Even in the resting state, the brain claims more than half of glucose usage. In this way, ketones are an effective way of using stored fats when the body is triggered to produce them, even before activity is added to lifestyle.[127] And, because of the fat-burning, hormonal, and metabolic shifts that facilitate ketosis within the body's systems, the metabolic rate increases considerably during this time. Additionally, because ketones offer minimal inflammatory byproducts in comparison to glucose, the brain operates better on them, which is why increased cognitive lucidity often accompanies low-carb diets and intermittent fasts. At the eighteen-hour mark of fasting, ketone production increases to the point that these agents begin to act as hormone-like communicators throughout the body, alerting systems to take such measures as to "reduce inflammation and repair damaged DNA for example."[128]

By the twenty-four-hour mark of fasting, the previously mentioned stage of autophagy has initiated.[129] As cells and tissues are rejuvenated and replaced with newer, healthier cells, immunity is increased and mental clarity continues to improve as a result of operating off ketones rather than glucose. Since growth hormone is secreted as a byproduct of ghrelin, the hunger-sensing hormone, an increasingly insatiate appetite over this moderate period of time lends to the increase of this beneficial hormone, which encourages lean tissue health, boosts cardiovascular health, and diminishes fat accumulation and storage. By the time you have been fasting for forty-eight hours, your "growth hormone level is up to five time as high" as it was before you started the fast.[130] When you've been food-deprived for fifty-four hours, insulin will be nearing a type of "reset" point, meaning that the body has adapted its insulin process to become more insulin-sensitive, and thus less insulin-resistant.[131] This helps decrease inflammation, along with arming your system with protective measures against such ailments as chronic disease, diabetes, and even cancer.

At the seventy-two-hour mark, autophagy hits an all-new level. On a cellular plain, IGF-1 (insulin-like growth factor 1) and PKA (protein kinase A) activity subsides. These two agents assure the life and growth of individual cells—regardless of their health—and thus inhibit autophagy. Considering that these elements exist to ensure that individual cells thrive, their inhibition may sound counterproductive, until we factor in the idea that these elements promote growth, division, and reproduction *even in unhealthy, degenerate, or maladaptive cells.* "PKA is the key gene that needs to shut down in order for…stem cells to switch into regenerative mode," and, IGF-1 is a "growth-factor hormone…linked to aging, tumor progression and cancer risk."[132] By depriving the body of food for a prolonged time, these agents are subdued; thus, individual cellular survival is forfeited for the sake of overall, uniform cellular health throughout the entire body.

During moderate to advanced stages of autophagy (when the body has fasted for seventy-two hours or more), your body additionally begins the miraculous process of replacing cells within the immune system. Not only are dead and degenerate cells throughout the rest of the body being replaced with newer, healthier ones, but immune cells are actually undergoing the process as well. This springs from the fact that stem cells are renewed and white blood cells flourish, something many studies have linked to being beneficial for those who have recently undergone or are still undergoing chemotherapy. While chemotherapy has long been regarded as a lifesaving tool for many patients, doctors also acknowledge the wreckage it places on the immune system. However, "prolonged fasting for 72 hours has been shown to preserve healthy white blood cell or lymphocyte counts in patients undergoing chemotherapy."[133]

So, how does autophagy rejuvenate the immune system? "White blood cells, also known as leukocytes, are the cells which the immune system uses to fight against foreign invaders like viruses and bad bacteria."[134] When we experience moderate periods of food deprivation, studies show that the hematopoietic stem cell system—a vital element of the immune system that is responsible for the health of blood and immune cells, but which is diminished in immunocompromised patients, such as those undergoing chemotherapy—hits a sort of reset button.[135] Studies with mice have shown that this process "has implications for chemotherapy tolerance and for those with a wide range of immune system deficiencies, including autoimmunity disorders."[136] This means that not only does the body have the potential to overcome current illness, but the system with the ability to prepare for and ward off future sickness is rearmed, having been given a complete overhaul.

When the body has fulfilled a seventy-two-hour fast, old, dead, dying, or degenerate tissues are being broken down and absorbed—replaced with fresh, healthier material. The immune system has been cleaned and rejuvenated. The entire physiology is cleansed, refreshed, and ready to defend against incoming agents of destruction; insulin sensitivity v. resistance is more balanced; metabolic rate is reset at a higher (faster) level; and the cognitive abilities of the mind are revitalized.

A quick Google search of the subject of healing while fasting renders hundreds of stories claiming miraculous healing during such an endeavor. I (Joe) prayed many times with a friend who went through a very difficult season after being diagnosed with a terminal brain tumor. After following an intermittent fasting regime that spanned more than two years, he announced that his body had "eaten" the tumor he had been battling. I'm certainly not claiming that everyone who practices intermittent fasting will experience a reversal of this magnitude, but I *am saying* that all levels of healing become possible when we submit, 100 percent, to all measures of healthy practices in our ardent search for God's will.

Jesus' Fasting

In religious circles, fasting is a period designated for complete or partial abstinence from food or other nutrients to appeal to God in a prayerful way. We see in Matthew 4 that, after He was baptized, Jesus was led by the Holy Spirit into the wilderness in order to fast for forty days and nights. Toward the end of this time, the devil tempted Him by exploiting His bodily desires, testing His level of authority, and even challenging His identity as the Son of God. After Jesus resisted the devil's persuasions, angels nourished Him (Matthew 4:11). He had fasted for an unprecedented length of time while facing these temptations. However, during His conversation with Satan, Jesus continually refuted the wiles of His foe by referring to Scripture, beginning His rebuttals with, "It is written…" (Matthew 4: 4, 7). In this way, Jesus set the example for us: In our ultimate weakness (in His case, having gone forty days with no nutrition), our strength and healing are found in the Lord. While fasting may, at times, make us feel as though our flesh is being weakened, our spirit gains strength when we deprive our flesh of its needs. Fasting isn't only a medically beneficial practice, but, as stated in *Timebomb*, it's a spiritual strengthener as well:

[Scripture tells us not to be] given to our fleshly desires, but… [to transcend] to a place where we look to Him to meet our needs. The desires of the flesh are often misconstrued as being merely sexual, but this isn't always true. The desires of the flesh include anything finite that keeps us from following the will of God. When we are fatigued, sluggish, or ineffective, our discernment cannot be sharpened. To truly surrender to the will of God is to follow Him in all our ways. Especially in light of the knowledge that many of us are biologically addicted to food, this heightens the alarm that our food is a combatant that we must arm ourselves against.[137]

The ironic thing about this is that, across the centuries since these passages were written, mankind has had a spiritual understanding of the stronghold of gluttony and the supernatural, deliverance-rendering power of fasting. However, only recently has science shown how making sacrifices of fleshly satisfaction can bring about healing on a medical level. These principles are confirmed by studies indicating that fasting rejuvenates every part of the body, clearing the mind of chemical inhibitors that slow cognitive ability while revitalizing the immune system, blood, organs, and other tissues by cleansing them of old, degenerate cells and supplying them with fresh, healthy ones.

It is also stated throughout Scripture that God *expects* us to fast:

"Therefore also now," saith the Lord, "turn ye even to me with all your heart, with fasting, and weeping, and with mourning." (Joel 2:12)

In the same way the body moves into a type of self-preservation mode when fasting, operating to rejuvenate and safeguard the body with a sense of urgency, the spirit, likewise, adopts a senses of determination when we fast. We are aware that, during a fast, the cellular level of the body is engaged in a type of preparation-preservation. It's interesting that fasting is a way of bringing the physical body into the same heightened spiritual plane of rejuvenation and rebirth that the mind enters while the flesh is being denied:

Fasting is calculated to bring a note of urgency and importunity to our praying, and to give force to our pleading in the court of heaven. The man who prays with fasting is giving heaven notice that he is truly in earnest.... He is using a means that God has chosen to make his voice be heard on high.[138]

Word of Caution

Intermittent fasting can be confused for a diet, since many people lose weight over the course of its practice, but it's really more about adopting a nutritional pattern than it is about ruling out certain foods while promoting others. With all this discussion of the health benefits that occur around the seventy-two-hour mark of fasting, you may be thinking that we're proposing that you immediately stop eating for at least three days.

That is *not* what we're suggesting.

In some circumstances, you should not attempt to fast without consulting a natural healthcare practitioner for guidance. Some who suffer medical conditions such as diabetes, poor blood-sugar regulation, or blood-pressure issues; who are severely underweight or have *ever* struggled with eating disorders who are pregnant, breastfeeding, attempting to conceive, or struggling with irregular menstrual cycles; or who are on regular prescription medications may be told that they should either avoid fasting altogether or engage in short durations of deprivation at most.

While the health benefits of moderate to prolonged fasting periods are certainly appealing, those with doubts *of any kind* regarding their medical response to the practice should seek the advice of a professional.

Additionally, fasting is a practice that takes practice. Sound redundant? That's because it's necessary to stress that the seventy-two-hour fast is a goal *we must work up to.* Many may believe that they're "tough enough" to take it on in one swoop, but they may be unaware of certain nutritional deficiencies that could cause a sudden attempt at such a long fast to be dangerous. The body needs time to adjust to such practices. With this said, for those who do decide to consider fasting, allow us to give some thoughts on how to initiate the habit.

How To Go About It

First of all, as stated, if you have a medical condition that could compromise your health when fasting, it's vital that you consult a natural healthcare professional. As mentioned, some who fast regularly may declare that they do so for days on end, which can be intimidating to those who are considering it for the first time. Important to remember is to ease into it, slowly. For example, if you're used to eating all hours of the day and night, your first step could be to take on a 12:12 (twelve-hour by twelve-hour) fasting schedule. This means that for twelve hours of the day, you'll refrain from food intake of any kind. So, if you eat breakfast at 8 a.m., then you should eat nothing after 8 pm.

It is generally accepted that coffee, green tea, and lemon/lime water are permissible during a fast, as long as you consume them in moderation. I (Joe) have found that green tea in particular helps tremendously with feelings of weakness or hunger during extended fasts. Herbal teas containing any fruit are not allowed, as many contain sugar that spikes insulin and ends the fast. You can drink water with healthy salt to keep the adrenal glands healthy during this time.

Once you've become accustomed to this schedule, you can transfer to a 14:10 regimen, meaning that all your eating must take place within a ten-hour period of each day. So, a breakfast at 8 a.m. will bring a dinner conclusion at 6 p.m. As you adapt to this, you can kick it up a notch by implementing a sixteen-hour fast (16:8). You can do this by eating an early dinner, followed by a late breakfast the next morning. This will be fairly simple, because it's likely that you'll be asleep for a large part of the fast. When you've had success at this, begin to implement your fasting twice a week. On one of the two days each week, narrow the eating hours on the day before a sixteen-hour fast, until you can convert it to a twenty-four-hour duration. After mastering this, work on the second sixteen-hour fast each week, until the practice has become two periods of twenty-four hours per week (from dinner that first day to dinner on the second day).

Eventually, you can take on the habit of eating an even earlier dinner on the day before a twenty-four-hour fast, followed by a later breakfast on the day following, which extends this period to thirty-six hours. As you continue to reduce your eating hours before or after the fast, the window of time you won't be consuming anything will eventually stretch to seventy-two hours. However, as stated already, a don't attempt to fast this long until you've have become thoroughly acquainted with how fasting impacts your body.

After the seventy-two-hour mark, additional health benefits occur and are worth looking into for anyone wishing to pursue more intense fasting. However, we're more interested in helping you reach a realistic level, which will benefit those who are struggling with illness or looking to boost overall health. For that reason, we won't discuss fasting longer than the three-day duration.

Another important—and commonly overlooked—element of fasting is re-introducing food into the system. Many people, motivated by elevated hunger sustained over a long period of time, follow a fast by succumbing to the seduction of overeating, indulging in gratuitous simple carbs, or even taking in toxic foods, presuming them to be justified in wake of their recent sacrifice for better health. Not only is this counterproductive, but it also throws off the system off as it reacclimates to the higher level of nutritional intake.

The food eaten at the end of a fast should be healthy, balanced, and organic. The diet should include complex carbohydrates (preferably from vegetables) in balance with proteins. When reintroducing food to the system, enteroendocrine cells in the gut release GLP1 (glucagon-like peptide 1) into the blood, which keep insulin balanced as the body readjusts to the nutritional intake.[139] If this influx is restored at a slow and steady pace, rather than in a spiking surge, GLP1 will remain in balance so it can then enter the brain's chemistry and help maintain improved cognitive function and insulin management by "act[ing] directly on neurons to promote synaptic plasticity, enhance cognition and bolster cellular stress resistance."[140]

By spending time and effort on recreating your eating patterns, you'll likely more carefully scrutinize *what* you eat as well. After all, to take such ownership of your diet will inspire you to ramp up the quality of what you're eating as well. We'll discuss how to go about that in an upcoming chapter.

How Long? That's Between You and God

Ultimately, when, how often, and the length of your fast are completely between you and God. We simply want to make you aware of the vast spiritual and physical benefits of adopting the practice. Further, the correlation between the seventy-two-hour mark and myriad seemingly miraculous health profits becomes our motivation for encouraging those who are physically able to fast to do so. However, we also understand that many readers may have complicated health issues that keep them from being able to fast that long.

If other health issues do prevent you from such an extreme fast, you have other options. For example, you might be able to miss one meal at a time, or you might choose one item to abstain from—such as coffee or a particular snack. Similarly, a modified version of intermittent fasting is known as the 5:2 method, wherein you can consume "500–600 calories on two non-consecutive days of the week, but eat normally the other 5 days."[141] This may be a good option for those whose doctors have warned against fasting altogether.

Even if you're unable to engage in long-term fasting, we want to encourage you by saying this: Any effort you make will be seen and honored by God.

Conclusion

As stated, *when* we do things can be as vital as *what* we do where questions of health are concerned. While many people are ready to recognize a type of "internal clock," few understand the function of the circadian rhythm and what it means to overall well-being. While taking sleep, activity, and nutrition seriously can lead to better health, understanding the timing of those three subjects *as well as how they interact with each other* provides a world of benefits as well. In upcoming chapters, we'll discuss these themes at greater length.

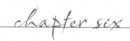
Sleep

In this chapter, we'll point out some surprising connections between sleep and vital body functions. We tend to vastly underappreciate the contribution sleep makes to our overall health. If we feel tired, we drink some coffee. Because we no longer feel tired, we don't realize that our bodies are still functioning under the compromised health that accompanies deprivation. This deficiency manifests in both physical and psychological ways. Further, when we feel we don't have enough time in our days, rather than cutting back on commitments to allow proper rest time, we often wake up earlier or "burn the midnight oil" to compensate for our busy lifestyles. In truth, we should be sleeping through one-third of our lives.

Often, we don't realize how important sleep is for our bodies' *vital (life-preserving) functions*. However, within every metric we use to assess our health, the only common denominator in one way or another is rest. It should seem more obvious when we consider that our bodies are made to shut off on their own if we neglect this necessity. Unfortunately, this mechanism can lead to other problems, ranging from students falling asleep in class to drivers passing out at the wheel and causing a fatal car accident (consequently, many doctors and scientists are now equating driving while sleep-deprived with driving under the influence of alcohol[142]). So, in considering the body's natural mechanism that mandates slumber even when we don't wish to prioritize it, that may come as a small surprise. Studies show that going two or three weeks without sleep, could be fatal.[143] More practically speaking, a study released in 2009 by Dr. Thomas Roth, director of research for sleep disorders at the Henry Ford Health System, stated that "chronic sleep restriction is associated with…a deterioration of daytime performance, including memory, and a number of physiologic consequences, including adverse effects on endocrine functions and immune responses and an increase in the risk of obesity and diabetes."[144] Sleep deprivation has also been correlated to type 2 diabetes, heart disease, obesity, and even premature death amongst the elderly.[145]

Grab Some Coffee?

Some think that the only bad effect of sleep deprivation is waking up tired. So, they believe creating a habit of morning caffeine intake equals problem solved.

No drowsiness, no problem—right?

Wrong!

Many don't realize that caffeine is a way of tricking your body into muting signals sent by something called adenosine—also referred to as "sleep pressure."[146] This is the substance that builds up within the brain during waking hours in order to induce sleep at the right times of the evening, and ensuring that sleep will last long enough to produce healing and restoration for the body and mind.

Caffeine, on the other hand, silences the signals sent by adenosine, kicking in about a half hour after consumption and staying in the system for between five to seven hours.[147] Thus, in addition to the damage done by lack of sleep because caffeine tricks us into thinking that we're not tired, caffeine gives us the added damage of adenosine being unable to lull us into slumber when it's finally time to sleep if we drink it too late in the day, as many do. The University of California at Berkeley's professor of neuroscience, Matthew Walker, stated that caffeine is "the most widely used (and abused) psychoactive stimulant in the world… [constituting] one of the longest and largest unsupervised drug studies ever conducted on the human race."[148]

During our waking hours, as stated previously, adenosine mounts within the brain—hence the phrase "sleep pressure"—until we rest and the pressure is relieved. We must achieve adequate amounts of this inactivity in order to remove all the mounted pressure, which builds in proportion to our waking hours. Sleep pressure carries over, meaning that long-term deprivation is accompanied by a continual, lingering amount of adenosine. This unrelieved burden feeds long-term sleepiness and fatigue, and even takes an overall toll on cognitive functions. While caffeine may temporarily alleviate the symptoms of the mounting adenosine, the sensation of sleep pressure will return as the caffeine wears off. There is only one way to be completely rid of this mounting compression: getting the proper amount of good-quality slumber.[149]

Unfortunately, many of us go about our days stifling the signal receptors of adenosine and "running on coffee." In doing so, we sell ourselves—and our health—short. This is often because we take sleep for granted, presuming that our brains are inactive while we sleep since we don't *remember* doing anything. However, nothing could be farther from the truth. In actuality, our brains are extremely busy while we sleep, conducting and overseeing an array of vital functions, without which our physical and psychological health are compromised.

Unfortunately, this is added to the before-mentioned fact that many are using technology too late in the day, allowing screen light to throw off their circadian rhythm and adversely impacting sleep routines. This further compromises our health via lack of quality and quantity of sleep. In fact, the National Sleep Foundation states that 90 percent of Americans regularly subject themselves to excessive screen time.[150] This negatively alters the structure of patterns that have evolved over the ages, exposing us to durations of light known by no previous generation.

Sleep Phases or Cycles

In beginning our study of sleep, we need to understand what the ideal night looks like and what cycles it includes. The ordinary sensory perceptions we notice during waking hours still surround us; our bodies can still feel, smell, and even taste while we're asleep. However, these signals don't usually pull us from slumber because the thalamus (the part of the brain that regulates signals of sensation) shuts off these triggers while we're asleep. The thalamus acts as a "gatekeeper," deciding which signals are worth interrupting sleep for and which to disregard.[151] As the body slips into sleep, there are multiple phases of sleep that we need to experience for quality rest. If the sleep cycle is interrupted or the body can't reach the full depth of each cycle, the brain is unable to complete the cycles of healing and detoxification that need to take place. Opinions vary as to how many phases take place in sleep. Some say the number is three: NREM (non-rapid eye movement), slow wave sleep, and REM (rapid eye movement). Others break down the stages further, rendering up to five. I, myself (Daniel), believe there are four: two phases of NREM, slow wave, and REM. Regardless, the operations that take place during sleep and their vitality remain the same. The entire sleep cycle lasts approximately ninety minutes and restarts throughout the night after each full rotation. Let's look at an example of a four-sleep-cycle model listed below:

NREM 1: The person has fallen into a light sleep. He or she is easily roused from this state, and if awakened, may be unable to tell whether sleep was achieved at all. This usually lasts only fifteen to twenty minutes.

NREM 2: The body is preparing for deep sleep. Muscles contract and unwind, but slowly settle into deeper relaxation as the body temperature decreases and the heart rate slows. This lasts approximately fifteen minutes.

Slow-wave sleep: This is sometimes also known as NREM 3. During this time, the brain is conducting metabolic, healing, and detox functions and effectively moving the previous day's memories into long-term memory storage. Muscle tissue is rejuvenated, the immune system is restored, and 95 percent of the daily supply of growth hormones is produced.[152] This can last up to an hour at a time.

REM: This phase usually lasts the final ten minutes of the sleep cycle. This is the when dreams take place, causing the eyes to move about under closed eyelids. REM concludes the sleep cycle, meaning that the full rotation of ninety-minute rest has been achieved. At this point, the body often stirs lightly and then reenters NREM1, restarting the succession. Ideally, we will experience four completed sequences each night for optimum health.

Growth Hormone

You might be thinking that human growth hormone is of no concern since you are a full-grown adult. However, while actual growth is part of "growth hormone's" appropriate context where children are concerned, the term also covers a vast array of processes that have nothing to do with reaching the physical adult size. These hormones stimulate "bone growth, immune function, amino acid uptake, protein synthesis and muscle glucose uptake," induce the "burning of fat from adipose tissues," and play a "key role in maintaining cardiovascular health."[153]

In other words, these are *very* important to the body's health. Thus, the deprivation of sleep that contributes to decline exacerbates health problems that stem from these systems reacting adversely through such responses as a weakened immune system, inefficient burning of fat, diminished muscle mass and performance, and increased signs of aging, such as thinning skin resulting in wrinkles.

Insulin

When most people think about certain lifestyle factors that affect insulin sensitivity and blood glucose levels, they think about nutrition, calories, fasting, or exercise. Sleep usually doesn't enter the conversation, because we rarely understand how vital sleep is to our blood sugar and glucose management. However, studies have shown a significant link between sleep deprivation and insulin sensitivity. Further, multiple nights of too little sleep can have negative long-term effects, including insulin resistance and impaired glucose tolerance. As a result, long-term sleep deprivation can lead to metabolic illness or conditions such as diabetes.

During slow-wave sleep, the growth hormone is produced and the nervous system's activity decreases. Additionally, the production of cortisol (a chemical that causes alertness and is often produced as a byproduct of stress) minimizes, which allows the brain to operate using less glucose, restoring glucose/insulin balance to the system.[154]

A lack of slow-wave sleep is related to such conditions as type 2 diabetes and other insulin-related illnesses. One study involved sleep disturbances that weren't intrusive enough to wake the participants, but were enough to keep them from lapsing into slow-wave sleep. After regularly practicing this for a series of nights, the participants were found to have 25 percent lower glucose tolerance (the body's ability to successfully process glucose) than before the experiment began. Another study showed that otherwise healthy people who were restricted to four to six hours of sleep each night for less than a week, like those in the previously mentioned study, marked a glucose tolerance that was lowered by an average of 40 percent, "reaching levels that are typical of older adults at risk for diabetes, which is characterized by high glucose levels due to insufficient insulin."[155] Further, when participants were fed breakfast, their glucose levels remained higher than their pre-experimental state, confirming the connection between glucose intolerance and sleep deprivation.[156] Lack of adequate rest has also been found to manifest in chronic stressing of the entire body, which contributes to elevated blood sugar as well, expounding the problem.[157]

In preparation for the morning, the body begins to secrete hormones that help us wake. This usually occurs between 3 and 4 a.m. The secreted hormones include growth hormones and cortisol, along with elevated blood sugar. These are the brain's way of preparing the body for a day of alertness and manual labor, but can result in overly heightened blood sugar upon waking for those who struggle with insulin imbalance, glucose tolerance, or diabetes.[158]

Snoring and Sleep Apnea

Unfortunately for those who have trouble getting a good night's rest due to snoring or sleep apnea, allowing the issue to go unaddressed can result in "developing certain types of metabolic syndrome(s); including diabetes, obesity, and high blood pressure. This likelihood…increased dramatically to 80% in those who found it difficult to fall asleep and to 70% for those who woke up not feeling as refreshed."[159] This is because those who chronically snore or suffer sleep apnea may have trouble reaching the deepest states of sleep, and thus are deprived of the "insulin reset" that takes place during slow-wave sleep. As an added frustration, chronic sleep deprivation can throw off blood sugar levels, causing them to elevate, which interferes with the body's ability to sleep. This creates a perpetuating cycle—and likewise elevates the risk of diabetes.[160]

Sleep disturbances can cause the overproduction of cortisol. Since this anti-inflammatory agent is the brain's response to stress, a little of it is beneficial. As stated earlier, *some* of this hormone is released in anticipation of waking up, to help us approach the incoming day with alertness. However, an overabundance (triggered by a brain that keeps waking throughout the night, as if in "false-start" motion) leads to obesity, reduced glucose tolerance, a weakened muscular and skeletal system, potentially high blood pressure, and worse, loss of cognitive function.[161]

Frequent Urination and Thirst

High blood sugar causes the kidneys to over-function, causing individuals to wake up many times throughout the night to urinate. This can be because the body is working too hard to expel elevated levels of sugar in the blood stream. Unfortunately, this can be another self-perpetuating issue, as interrupted sleep feeds chronic sleep deprivation, which in turn increases glucose levels. In response, the body craves water to support the continual urination, triggering more sleep disruptions and excess fluids that the body will attempt to expel. Again, the cycle can continue if not addressed.[162]

Obesity

Ghrelin is a hormone that triggers the "hungry" mechanism in our brain. Leptin—its partner in crime—dispatches in tandem with it, often sending out a sensation similar to panic to our brains, convincing us that we are starving. Unfortunately, sleep deprivation causes production of ghrelin to increase by as much as 15 percent, causing our hunger to spike. Leptin is thrown completely out of balance, adding an urgency to the hunger that is felt by the sleep-deprived snacker. Simultaneously, metabolism slows alongside the fat-burning mechanism, causing the body to consume more calories and store more fat than it is able to burn in a day. The cycle can lead to obesity; those who get less than four hours of rest habitually increase their odds of becoming obese by 73 percent.[163]

Cardiovascular Health

Because of the strong correlations between hypertension, high blood pressure, diabetes, heart attack, stroke, and obesity, it seems obvious that cardiovascular health is greatly affected by our sleeping habits. But recently, studies are confirming a direct link between "preclinical atherosclerosis [hardening of arteries as a byproduct of plaque] and…a higher rate of death among patients with heart disease."[164] Dr. Arshed Quyyumi, director of the Emory Clinical Cardiovascular Research Institute, oversaw the analysis of data from more than 2,800 coronary artery disease patients revealing that nearly 80 percent of those studied had an increased risk of mortality and simultaneously slept either under or above the recommended timeframe for nightly rest.[165] Factoring in variables, the doctor concluded that there was "almost a 40 to 50% increased risk of dying if you are sleeping too little or too much."[166]

Atherosclerosis, as mentioned before, is plaque buildup in arteries that, over time, causes them to harden. In one study, experimenters segregated two groups of mice and treated them just the same, other than keeping one group awake while the others were allowed ample sleep. The rest-deprived mice underwent a plummet in their levels of hypocretin—a hormone in the hypothalamus that promotes the "awake" feelings enjoyed by those who practice healthy sleeping habits. Similarly, in patients who have sleep disorders such as narcolepsy, hypocretin is unusually low. The decreasing presence of this substance in the mice caused the body to respond with a spike in a protein known as CSF1, which "increased production of inflammatory white blood cells in the bone marrow and accelerated atherosclerosis."[167] Conversely, when hypocretin levels were again balanced within the mice, the atherosclerosis process immobilized.[168]

Because atherosclerosis can lead to stroke, hypertension, heart attack, and coronary artery disease, and can affect nearly all the major organs of the body, this imbalance of hormones can be a dire, even deadly, threat. This is just one more way that regular sleep helps regulate the balance of hormones and other body chemicals and keeps inflammation—and many chronic illnesses—at bay.

Cognitive Function and Emotional Well-being

Poor sleep can impair cognitive functions in many ways. While some may seem as simple as grumpiness or irritability, others are more severe, including disruption of "concentration, alertness, and reflexes, making sleep-deprived individuals more prone to falls and accident-related injury."[169] Recent studies have shed additional light on the nature of sleep as it pertains to psychological health: While previous generations perceived sleeping disorders to be a result of psychiatric disorders, the reverse is now being understood to be true. In other words, while medical and psychological professionals used to think psychological misalignments fostered poor sleep, they now believe that chronic sleep disturbances encourage psychological imbalances.[170] In fact, at this time, there is not a single known psychiatric disorder that doesn't have an accompanying sleep disorder.

The *Oxford Academic Journal* released the results of a study wherein fifty-six otherwise healthy high-school-aged teens were subject to a short series of nights in which sleep was incrementally reduced until the duration reached only five hours per night. The subjects were otherwise academically proficient students performing at top-rated high schools. The nights with a five-hour sleep limitation were then maintained for a series of seven nights. Those deprived of full-length sleep immediately began to show decreased ability to perform academically, along with "deterioration in sustained attention, working memory and executive function, increase in subjective sleepiness, and decrease in positive mood."[171] The results of the study revealed that even just a week of sleep deprivation "impairs a wide range of cognitive functions, subjective alertness, and mood" for top-level performing students who, even after two nights of recovery sleep, still manifested such symptoms.[172] In a separate, similar study, subjects likewise manifested these symptoms along with delayed reaction times (another contributor to dangerous driving, as mentioned earlier)—and worse, after fourteen days of this practice, they didn't report feeling especially sleepy.[173] What's alarming about this is the fact that, despite the body's willingness to attempt to adapt to the lack of sleep, the underlying health consequences remain.

Sleep likewise facilitates the storage of memories accrued over the course of the day, which are temporarily stored in the hippocampus during waking hours. The hippocampus is the part of the brain that saves all incoming information until slow-wave sleep occurs, during which the information is consolidated and moved into the brain's cortex. This data is then stored as long-term memories, or "learned information." While adequate sleep is vital for people of all ages, the fruits of sleep deprivation can be particularly observed in young adults. Those who stay up late "cramming" for a test will likely receive less benefit than those who study in advance and then get a good night's rest the night before the exam. Not only will the information be more reliably stored within the brain, but the decreased level of anxiety (because of adequate rest and the knowledge having been securely stored and accessible) will allow the brain to perform better as well.

On the other hand, many experts believe the hippocampus has a limited time for hanging on to new information—a sort of expiration date. If information isn't preserved by being purged and sent to the cortex within a set amount of time (experts currently estimate about sixteen hours), the information can become distorted or disappear altogether.[174]

Thus, chronic disruption of sleep interrupts the formation of new memories and the ability to learn. Because this transfer is completed during the slow-wave sleep phase, it is vital to get quality, *deep* sleep every night. The lack of this kind of sleep is a large contributor to cognitive impairment among the elderly; experts note a link between slow-wave sleep and "age-related medial prefrontal cortex (mPFC) gray-matter atrophy."[175] In plain English, brains deprived of slow-wave sleep for long periods can begin to malfunction where memory storage is concerned, leading to the brain's inability to store and maintain memories.[176] This sheds an entirely new light on ailments such as Alzheimer's disease, which is accompanied by cognitive decline. In fact, a prequel to this illness is often chronic sleep disturbance, since it encourages the production of a degenerative protein called amyloid-beta, which collects in the prefrontal cortex, forming plaque and promoting the development of Alzheimer's.[177] "The severity of accumulation significantly predicts the degree and extent of cognitive decline associated with Alzheimer's."[178] In turn, amyloid-beta contributes to sleep deprivation, perpetuating the cycle.[179] During normal slow-wave sleep, the brain is purged of up to 40 percent of this substance, thanks to the glymphatic system.[180]

As the body encounters slow-wave sleep, the glymphatic system—a perivascular system that supports the blood vessels supplying the brain—rids the brain of toxins and waste, sending a rush of fluids that clear away "proteins and metabolites from the central nervous system" by expanding, essentially squeezing out toxins and then diminishing once again, creating space for the brain's blood flow to again move freely, rejuvenating it.[181] This system is responsible for distributing beneficial substances to the brain, such as "essential nutrients such as glucose, lipids…amino acids…growth factors and neuromodulators."[182]

At this point, you may assume that these cognitive problems resulting from insufficient sleep are limited to the elderly, but allow us to assure you that this is not so. It can affect people as young as those in their late twenties.[183] For some of these younger adults, snoring, sleep apnea, or other illness may contribute to this deprivation, but for a vast majority, the real culprit is lifestyle. Studies have shown that a sleep destitute period lasting up to thirty-six hours can instigate an increase in the level of amyloid-beta up to 30 percent.[184]

In addition to affecting the storing and facilitating of our memories, our sleep schedules also vastly influence our mood. We then carry these influences into our lifestyles, affecting our overall happiness and quality of life, which disturbs sleep, feeding a vicious cycle. Recent studies have revealed what is becoming known as a "phenotype of social withdrawal and loneliness," meaning that sleep disturbance contributes to neural and behavioral components that can be picked up on by peers and that cause us to remain withdrawn from social interaction.[185] The result is isolation, which, in turn, contributes to loneliness and sleep disturbance, feeding the sequence. Those who suffer this cycle additionally see increased odds of "cardiovascular disease, alcoholism and suicidality, physical diseases related to stress and compromised immune function, and in later life, greater risk of degenerative dementia,"[186] while altering behavior and emotions…also disturbing essential metabolic processes and influencing the expression of immune-related genes."[187]

Having belabored the point already that, in order to enjoy good health, we must have social interaction, community, and quality of life, we will not linger here; this point speaks for itself.

The Importance of Melatonin

For many, sleep disruption is related to reduced melatonin production as we age.[188] But melatonin is not just a sleep drug. It is responsible for many other functions, such as "regulating the neuroendocrine system… metabolism, sex drive, [and] appetite."[189] Likewise, it prevents rapid reproduction of cancer cells and fortifies the immune system via its antioxidant properties.[190] It is said that by the time we reach the age of sixty, our melatonin production is nearly dormant in the evening hours. By age eighty, melatonin is nearly undetectable in the system. This correlation is significant, because as we note how many health problems occur as a result of poor sleep, we can see a spike in these same issues amongst the elderly. In fact, studies have shown that chronic sleep deprivation can actually increase the odds of premature death among seniors by 100 percent (X2).[191] If we were able to ensure better, *deeper* sleep for these individuals, they would likely enjoy greater health into later years of their lives.

Inflammation

Cytokines is a generalized term that refers to "small secreted proteins released by cells [that] have a specific effect on the interactions and communications between cells."[192] When the length of sleep is shortened, our bodies secrete pro-inflammatory cytokines (which can include but are not limited to C-reactive protein or CRP, IL-6, and IL-17) within the body that are able to act on either the very cells that disbursed them, or on nearby or even distant ones.[193] A solid connection has been established between certain pro-inflammatory cytokines and chronic pain via "nociceptive sensory neurons,"[194] otherwise known as pain receptors. In other words, when we are sleep deprived, our bodies secrete chemicals that move directly to our pain sensors—and this manifestation can be sporadic throughout the body—and instigate painful inflammation. If we wake up in pain, it is likely that we did not sleep well, and the body responded by secreting pro-inflammatory triggers in anticipation of pain or stress, ironically self-inflicting the anticipated discomfort upon itself. Studies have shown that CRP and IL-17 can remain in the body for more than two days past the time that normal sleep resumes.[195]

However, there is more to be concerned than just mere discomfort. Dr. Zack Bush asserts that chronic inflammation is actually at the origin of all chronic illness.[196] According to Bush, all disease, when scrutinized in its most microscopic form, is a byproduct of chronic inflammation.[197] With this in mind, it becomes apparent that the secretion of pro-inflammatory cytokines can be a large contributor to chronic illnesses, and these are fortified by sleep deprivation. Thus, one of the body's best defense systems can be found in getting plenty of rest.

How to Sleep Better

If you realize, after reading this chapter, that you haven't been getting enough sleep, there are steps you can take to rectify the issue. Recall our discussion in a previous chapter of lifestyle and choices. When you decide to change your ways for the sake of your health, you've already taken the first step. However, as mentioned, as we age, melatonin production diminishes, leaving many who would be willing to sleep unable to do so.

However, a determined person will find that there are many strategies to help alleviate this issue. You can begin to create space within your mind and schedule for the purpose of relieving anxiety at bedtime, and for allowing proper "wind-down" time before bed. It has been made clear by this point that our fast-paced lifestyle is counterproductive to inducing a healthy sleep schedule. So, it's important to work on slowing your pace in the hours approaching bedtime. Your home life *must* be peaceful and allow for respite. If you can't obtain *peace* in your setting of rest, surely you will be unable to achieve *sleep* just the same way. Remember that this is more than mental; hormonal secretions take place before bed, and they work best when they are able to follow circadian cues.

When we are experiencing stress (such as being worried about a hypothetical future, or reliving a past traumatic event), the brain reads the accompanying chemical responses just the same as if a life-threatening emergency were taking place. It is vital that we relinquish the worries of the day before we attempt to retire. This is why Philippians 4:6–7 tells us to "be anxious for nothing, but in everything by prayer and supplication, with thanksgiving, let your requests be made known to God; and the peace of God, which surpasses all understanding, will guard your hearts and minds through Christ Jesus" (NKJV).

We should limit participating in rigorous activities and taking in caffeine to earlier parts of the day. Ideally, we should engage in our heaviest physical activities in the hours *before* dinner. And, since caffeine can remain in the body for up to five to seven hours, if we must indulge in caffeine-loaded drink, the last one of the day we should have should be before lunch. As noted in our discussion of the circadian clock, if we don't time these activities in accordance with the body's rhythm, it will prevent melatonin and other necessary sleep-inducing functions to happen on target. On the same note, as explained previously, we should avoid snacking after dinner, as it will flip the body's "fat-burning switch" back and forth, in and out of time, throwing off quality and quantity of sleep.

Beyond deciding to relinquish worries before bed, there are other practical things you can do to help wind down at night. For example, limit exposure to blue light. As we've stated, we're exposed to light durations never known to previous generations, and which, quite frankly, aren't even natural. When the sun goes down, blue-light exposure in your home should diminish as well. Keep lamps low and read a book, knit, do a puzzle, or hold a conversation with a loved one. Resist the urge to allow electronic communication (such as texting or social media) to keep you engaged late into the evening. We recommend no screens of any kind (i.e., scrolling through social media on your phone) for at least a half-hour before bedtime.

A routine at bedtime helps significantly. It can be difficult to come home from a busy day and go straight to bed. This is because the mind's intellectual (not circadian) clock hasn't completely received communication that bedtime is indeed imminent. A routine provides a subliminal messaging system that trains your mind to recognize the approach of sleep time.

It doesn't need to be elaborate or expensive, but make sure your bed and bedroom are comfortable. If neatness is important to you, keep your bedroom clean. Make sure the room temperature is at an appropriate setting. Try to find a mattress comfortable enough that body pains don't disturb the quality of your sleep; and ensure that pillows and blankets are comfortable. See that the room is dark enough that you're able to drift off without trouble—and if noises bother you, try white noise such as a fan to drown it out.

Some find it helpful to make sure the bedroom is used only for sleeping. For example, I (Joe) have a friend who works from home, and for a short time, she attempted to work at a desk in her bedroom. However, when it was time to go to bed, the lingering stacks of undone work hovered too near, keeping her mind from being able to relinquish the day's unfinished responsibilities. When she moved the desk out of her bedroom, she began to sleep better. So, make sure that your bedroom is used only for activities that don't impede your ability to rest.

For years during the course of my medical issues, I (Joe) struggled with insomnia. If you try the suggestions we have made and still have problems getting to sleep, I'd like to share some solutions that have brought me relief. First, herbal teas consisting of chamomile, valerian root, lavender, lemon balm, or magnolia bark all work to increase or modify neurotransmitters that are involved in initiating sleep. Drinking a cup of one of these types of teas can be an inexpensive way to decrease nighttime awakenings and improve your overall sleep quality. Many brands offer a variety of blends of the aforementioned herbs, but I've found the most success with those that are organic, marketed specifically for sleep, and feature chamomile as the primary ingredient.

So, I've experienced significant success with herbal teas. However, *nothing has helped me achieve consistent REM sleep the way that CBD (cannabidiol) oil has.*

Unlike many of the over-the-counter and prescription sleep aids that often carry lengthy warning labels and side effects, CBD acts on receptors throughout the body known as the endocannabinoid system. CBD is non habit-forming, non-addictive, and an efficient way to fight insomnia and assure a deep, full cycle of sleep. It is also great as an anti-inflammatory agent, eases physical pain and anxiety, relaxes muscles, eliminates nightmares, and provides relief from psychological trauma-related conditions such as PTSD. We could literally write an entire book on the benefits of its healing properties, but for the purposes of this volume, here is an overview.

CBD is derived from the cannabis plant (*Cannabis sativa*), which sometimes causes people to shy away from its use. However, this is born out of a misconception that all cannabis products contain THC (tetrahydrocannabinol), the psychoactive element in cannabis that makes one feel "high" when using marijuana. However, cannabidiol is one of more than one hundred chemical compounds this plant produces.[198]

Many people assume that using CBD oil is the same as using marijuana, or that this product will make them lose control of their mental faculties or otherwise experience symptoms of drug use. However, that is not the case. The cannabis plant is actually very complex, and that renders many unique and valuable chemical elements. THC is a psychoactive compound, but CBD *is not.*[199] While many areas are experiencing rapidly changing laws regarding the recreational use of marijuana, few medical professionals deny its value for patients who cannot escape physical pain. Thus, there are provisions for its medical use. However, for some, this leaves the moral conundrum regarding whether God approves of its use as a pain modifier and sleep aid. Thus, many forego this treatment. This is understandable, as those who perceive God as one who wants us to "be sober and vigilant" (1 Peter 5:8) at all times have a moral conflict with the concept of taking something that could potentially make them high.

However, as noted previously, CBD is not a psychoactive like its counterpart, THC. With this being said, many have found relief similar to that offered by other elements of the cannabis plant, but without the properties that may cause concern regarding the moral issues. We'll discuss the use of CBD oil for chronic pain management in an upcoming chapter.

Finally, if sleep issues persist, you can consult a natural healthcare practitioner and see if they encourage the use of a melatonin supplement or other herbal solution. A professional will be able to note whether other culprits are contributing to sleeplessness, or even if another supplement will provide a better result.

chapter seven

Nutrition and Gut Health

We discussed earlier how modern farming practices have made it more difficult to obtain healthy food. Between chemicals sprayed on crops and the depletion of our soil through over-farming, even foods that pose as the healthiest can be devoid of nutrition.

Before we move on, let's take a minute to define nutrition. A nutrient is an agent that carries into the body a means of both survival and nourishment for thriving. It's primarily delivered to our bodies in the form of carbohydrates, proteins, and fats;[200] but other vehicles of nutrition are vitamins, minerals, fiber, water, and oxygen. Nutrients include two categories: micronutrients and macronutrients. The first category includes those we can live on small quantities of, while the second, the macros, are nutrients we require in larger measures. An example of a micronutrient is iron, while macronutrients include substances like water and protein.[201]

Modern Habits Sabotage Our Health

We face an ironic paradox. While our society has more access to food than many previous generations, we're more malnourished on average than those same ancestors. It seems odd that a populace with such wealth and abundant availability of food—and with such an obesity epidemic— would be suffering from deficiencies of some of the most basic nutrients. Yet, Dr. Zack Bush points out an "inverse relationship" between being well-nourished and obese.[202] ("Inverse" indicates "opposite": When one number goes down on a chart, the other one comes up, and vice versa). This is counterintuitive: You would think that an obese person would have no nutritional deficiencies because of plentiful access to food. However, this assumption hinges on the concept that obesity is caused by eating *large quantities of healthy food*, which is rarely the case these days. Many individuals are surprised to learn that their health problems stem from the fact that they are extremely undernourished.

In addition to the fact that our food is depleted of many of its nutrients, there is (again) the issue of circadian rhythm where sustenance is concerned. Recall that previous generations only had access to food for about twelve hours a day, because once it was dark outside, they didn't go out in pursuit of it. Many people only ate about two meals a day, and those who ate three didn't snack. Thus, nutrients were ingested in proportion to the body's rhythm and need, and didn't fight against the its systems. This allowed the physiology to fully absorb and benefit from the nourishment ingested.

Depletion of Nutrition

In 2004, the *Journal of the American College of Nutrition* published a report based on a USDA analysis comparing produce grown in 1950 and 1999. The results showed that produce appearing the same actually showed a vast decline in nutrients in just forty-nine years. For example, radishes saw a 50 percent decline in calcium and protein, a 10 percent drop in phosphorous, and a whopping 75 percent decrease in vitamin A. Tomatoes had fallen 15 percent in protein, 30 percent in ash, 45 percent in calcium, 12 percent in phosphorous, 25 percent in iron, and 50 percent in vitamin A. Kohlrabi dropped 20 percent in protein, more than 50 percent in calcium, nearly 10 percent in phosphorous, 44 percent in iron, 17 percent in thiamin, and 40 percent in riboflavin. Celery saw a loss of 60 percent in protein, 30 percent in fat, 25 percent in calcium, more than 60 percent in phosphorous, 20 percent in iron, and 20 percent in niacin. Radishes and tomatoes were diminished by 10 percent in ascorbic acid, which is a cofactor to vitamin C. These numbers may seem shocking, but they are only a few examples of how our produce has changed over the last several decades.

This has happened largely because, as soil is farmed too regularly with no time to replenish, each crop sponges more resources from the bankrupt ground. Soil ecology is vital to the nutritional value of our food, yet sadly has been left out of the equation far too many years. In turn, as discussed previously, the crops yield plants with less and less to offer in the way of nutrients. Even when fertilizer is used, often the result is an apple or a tomato that *looks* like the ones our grandparents ate, but that doesn't pack the same nutritional punch. When dangerous farming chemicals such as weed killers are added to the mix, we see a cruel conundrum: Those who are tricked into thinking they have taken the healthy route by purchasing fresh produce are still at risk of developing chronic illness.

Local, Organic Food

This is where the argument for locally grown, organically raised food becomes the most compelling option when it comes to eating for good health. These foods, obviously, are grown in nutrient-rich soil that hasn't been depleted by over-farming for several decades. Additionally—and, again, obviously—the organic methods of farming keep chemical exposure to a minimum. And the benefits of local, organic foods aren't limited to gardens, crops, and orchards; even when it comes to fresh meat, locally raised is best. (For further information on that, please see Joe's book, *Timebomb*, which covered the issue at length.)

There is another plus, however, to purchasing locally grown, organic food. Consider, for example, an apple. When you eat an apple that has been harvested in your area, it has survived and thrived by adapting to the environment, thus in a sense "inoculates" you with its benefits based on its own ecology. Think about it: The fruit or vegetable will have been farmed to strengthen you for thriving in your own environment and surroundings! Many understand how locally produced honey helps them deal with allergies: Bees use pollen from a specific region's plants to create the honey. When we eat that honey, then, our bodies receive small exposures to the properties of the pollen producers. In response, our bodies create proper response for the allergens—and we no longer suffer. This is an example of our own ecology feeding us *and* arming us against local hazards.

This is another reason our systems are sabotaged when we eat foods that have been shipped in from another country—or worse, sprayed with chemicals. Food, until it's removed from its life source, is, of course, living. Thus, it literally becomes stronger as it survives environmental hardships, and that strength is passed on to us. When we can step back to look at the bigger picture, we see that our indigenous location provides what we need to be healthy.

Additionally, when food is shipped in from other areas of the world, we have no way of knowing how long it was harvested before we eat it. This may seem insignificant, but let's look at the example of an apple again.

When we pull an apple from a tree, we cut it off from its life source, and it immediately starts to die. Every moment after that, the nutritional value is diminishing and waste is increasing proportionately (fruit's version of the same decomposition process that happens to everything that dies). Food industry practice is to modify the fruit so that it looks fresh (for example, by waxing the fruit), but regardless of cosmetic efforts, the apple is dead. When produce has been recently picked, it is safe and even beneficial to eat because it's early in the breakdown course. However, the rotting continues until, eventually, the fruit is no longer safe for consumption, and we throw it away. Often, eating something that is still merely "safe" (not rotten) isn't the same as saying it's still full of beneficial nutrients. When produce has been removed from its life source for a significant length of time, its nutrients died long before it reaches our kitchen countertop. We may *think* we're eating fresh fruit, but in actuality, we're eating dead waste.

Canned Food

Some people shy away from canned foods because of the added sugar. While we encourage everyone to minimize sugar intake, this concern can be misplaced. In earlier generations, when people primarily raised their own food, there was a period each year when no fresh food was available. That's why they preserved much of their harvest with sugar, salt, or fermentation. When food is canned (even though sugar is often added), it's placed in liquid that cuts off contact with oxygen. This arrests the decomposition process, because oxygen is what triggers the breakdown. In this way, canned, homegrown food—even containing sugar—can be healthier than eating produce purchased at a big-box grocery store. However, it is always best to avoid sugar when possible.

Fermentation

Fermentation, a process developed in the days before refrigeration, is a great way to preserve food—and it provides beneficial bacteria. In fact, it's one of the healthiest ways to take in nutrition, because the beneficial bacteria produced during fermentation promote healthy gut microbiota. Thus, the colon is replenished with healthy bacteria that fortifies personal ecology. The health and flora of the gut is one of the most vital ways we can boost immunity, fight chronic illness, and keep our bodily systems functioning properly (more on this in a bit).

Are You Malnourished?

It isn't hard to tell if you're malnourished. In fact, there are many symptoms, and they're easy to detect, including: fatigue; physical weakness; frequent illness; extended recovery time after illness or injury; difficulty focusing, remembering, or concentrating; feeling chilly when others are comfortable; experiencing emotional distress; and undergoing psychological or cognitive slumps.[203] The problem with such obvious signals is that they often go unaddressed under the presumption that they're "normal" since they are so common. Another way to know if you are struggling with a nutritional deficiency is as simple as noticing an improvement after you begin to take vitamins or supplements.

Also, because the symptoms of malnutrition are so commonplace, it's easy to assume that they're not red flags. However, just as stressed in *Timebomb*, these warning signs are the body's way of alerting you to problems. Left unaddressed, they will likely escalate. Even without proper nutrition, the body must continue its ordinary functions. As noted earlier, the RMR (resting metabolic rate) burns 75 percent of output in most people. This means that while you're unaware of the workload your body is carrying, it's nevertheless a machine that—even in its resting state—has an enormous output that it can't afford to "slide" on, because your life depends on it. Thus, when your body isn't getting the nutrition it needs, it will *look* within your systems for places from which to rob or borrow these resources. Or, it will deprive areas of the body that are trying to heal because it needs those nutrients for life-sustaining functions. Over time, "borrowing from Peter to pay Paul" depletes the physiology's systems and organs of essential nutrients and eventually compromises the immune system. The result is a body that's unable to fight chronic illness.

You can see why proper nutritional intake is necessary for survival.

How can we make sure that we are getting enough nutrients? The answer isn't found in some sort of miracle supplement that will answer all of our nutritional needs so we can keep eating toxic or nutrient-deficient food. The key is to contact a natural healthcare practitioner, who can assess our deficiencies and help us correct them through food or supplements. However, we should work to transition to getting any nutrients we're drawing from supplements to getting them directly from a food source as soon as possible. For many, the body has an extremely difficult time absorbing vitamins and minerals carried via pill, capsule, or powder.

Macros and Micros

At the beginning of the chapter, we briefly discussed that micronutrients are nutrients we can live on in smaller proportions, while macronutrients are those we need in larger quantities. It is critical that we take in both types of nutrients in the proper allotments. When we don't, key metabolic processes are disrupted, which interrupts healing processes and hinders the conversion of food to energy. This in turn suppresses our ability to burn calories, contributing to the storage of fats that otherwise could have been utilized. Furthermore, inflammation levels can be affected by micros and macros not being consumed in proper amounts, and chronic illness—again—has an opportunity to take root.

The three most commonly noted macronutrients are fats, proteins, and carbohydrates.

Fats

Many people have a notion that avoiding fats is healthy. This is because so many fats in our foods are toxic, and when their evils are exposed, the nontoxic fat—the proverbial "baby"—gets thrown out with the "bathwater." However, this is a devastating mistake. Fats are vital for brain health, and they assist in cell development and function, insulate and protect the body's organs, support hormone production and balance, and accommodate nutrition absorption. Healthy fats such as those found in walnuts and almonds, avocados and olives—to name just a few sources—should actually make up about 15 to 20 percent of our diet.[204]

Proteins

Meat is a source of protein, but it's not the only vehicle that carries this important macronutrient into the body. Beans, seeds, nuts, legumes, and high-quality fresh produce all have protein,[205] which helps the body produce, repair, and reconstruct a variety of tissues, such as bone, skin, and muscle. It also originates body chemicals such as hormones and enzymes.[206] Likewise, it provides amino acids, which are a huge contributor to the immune system.[207] Like fats, proteins should make up 15 to 20 percent of our daily caloric intake.

Carbohydrates

Like fat, carbohydrates have gotten a bad rap in recent years. Many who have successfully (or not so) lost weight during trendy, low-carb diets have embraced the concept that carbs equal excess body fat, thus are the enemy. This couldn't be farther from the truth—if we're discriminate about *what type of carbs* we take in. Generally speaking, there are two types of carbohydrates: complex and simple. The former are found in foods such as fruits, dairy, nuts, vegetables, and legumes, and are constructed mainly of fiber and starch.[208] Simple carbohydrates are made of sugar.[209] When the body takes in simple carbs, they are converted into sugar glucose, which is subsequently transformed to fat or burned as energy. Complex carbs digest more slowly and carry other elements, causing the body's processing function to use the energy more easily rather than defaulting to total storage as fat. Because the elements within the complex carb are converted more slowly, blood sugar is more easily regulated, showing fewer "spikes" and "crashes." Simple carbs, on the other hand, convert to glucose quickly, causing a roller-coaster of blood-sugar imbalance that can be particularly dangerous for those who have type 2 diabetes. We need the energy-providing, complex carbs to make up between 45–65 percent of our daily caloric intake.[210]

Micronutrients

Just because micronutrients are necessitated in smaller increments than the macros, they're not any less important to our health. On the contrary, micro deficiencies left unaddressed can be dangerous. Common deficiencies include iron, iodine, vitamin D, vitamin B-12, calcium, vitamin A, and magnesium.[211] (Note that many of these correlate with the examples given earlier of produce showing a marked depletion in nutrients since 1950). Shortages in these vitamins and minerals can cause anemia, fatigue, a weakened immune system, cognitive interruption, metabolic malfunction, impairment of brain function or detox, developmental abnormalities, muscle weakness, and bone degradation. Low supplies of these key elements in our systems can even increase the odds that we'll develop chronic illnesses or diseases such as cancer or Alzheimer's disease.[212]

It would seem that we could simply supplement our diets with micros to ensure we receive enough of them, but this can be dangerous. This is especially true with micros such as iron or potassium, and even more so for those who have underlying methylation/absorption issues (more on this in a moment). It is important to only take supplements when a physician or natural healthcare practitioner advises. This, again, is why we suggest addressing as many deficiencies as possible through modifications in the diet.

Essential Fatty Acids

You may have heard mention of "essential fatty acids." The phrase can seem confusing, since the word "essential" has a specific meaning in this context. In this case, it refers to the fact that the body literally will not operate without it: We *need* essential fatty acids to make and dispense hormones, form memories, and maintain metabolic function. These are *biologically necessary* for basic living.

So, exactly what are essential fatty acids? The body is usually able to convert incoming nutrition into fats, but it cannot manufacture them. We must take them in through diet. They also differ from other fats in that they aren't stored as energy, but instead perform other key roles. For example, they improve cognitive function and enhance neural communication, which defends against conditions such as ADHD (attention-deficit/hyperactivity disorder), combats anxiety and depression, stabilizes moods (even for patients with such conditions as bipolar disorder and schizophrenia), and increases memory storage.[213] As such, they reduce our risk of developing such degenerative diseases as Alzheimer's and Parkinson's.[214] They balance cholesterol levels between "good" and "bad" and lower blood pressure, thus improving cardiovascular health.[215] Likewise, they contribute to healthier and cleaner arterial walls, preventing blood clots and arterial plaque buildup. Essential fatty acids balance chemicals that contribute to inflammation, keeping this issue—even chronic inflammation—in check. Additionally, they've been shown to reduce liver fat, diminishing the risk of illness related to fatty liver (large amounts of fat stored in the liver).[216] They also help balance insulin, improve insulin resistance, and prevent type 2 diabetes.[217] Because they promote healthy communication amongst the signalers and receptors throughout the body and keep hormones and other chemicals balanced, they reduce the probability of acquiring autoimmune disease, and are even used for treatment in such conditions as "lupus, rheumatoid arthritis, ulcerative colitis, Crohn's disease and psoriasis."[218] Their role as agents of neural communication ensures hormone balance, which means an imbalance or deficiency of these elements can contribute to malfunction affecting the entire body. Essential fatty acids also have been correlated with a lower risk of cancer, elevated heart health, reduced aging, and even better-quality sleep.[219]

So how do we go about adding essential fatty acids to our diet? The answer is found in a variety of seafood, nuts, seeds, and plant (non-synthetic) oils such as avocado or flaxseed. By seeking out healthy fats, we can assure that we have an adequate supply of these life-giving elements.

Water

Water is a source of life and healing. Scripture places great importance on water. It is called the pure element that will wash our souls clean (Hebrews 10:22), the healing revival for a thirsty land (Isaiah 44:3), and a serene place where God guides and heals our souls (Psalm 23:2). We're told that God will fill us from His spring of life (Revelation 21:6), and that living water will be given to all who ask (John 7:38). With all this in mind, it isn't hard to understand that the Creator made water a significant life source for His creation.

Water is the largest single component of our bodies, acting as a primary building block of our cells, and accounting for 60 percent of the human makeup, with some organs, such as the lungs, consisting of as much as 83 percent water.[220] Water is unique in that it is actually a liquefied crystal. It is essential for every function that our bodies conduct, from digestion to metabolic processes and organ operations, to energy production, to hormonal production and balance, and even to skin and reproduction health. Nearly everyone knows that the quantity of water we take in directly affects our health, however, the *quality* of that water we consume is just as important.

While many of us think we must try to drink all the water our body needs, we often overlook the fact that food has water in it as well. By eating proper amounts of fresh foods, we consume myriad micronutrients that are delivered to our bodies alongside quality hydration. Taking in water via food is healthier for a few reasons. First, water in our food carries vitamins and minerals to the bloodstream, which helps us better absorb the nutrients. Second, water in its natural source—such as in a tomato or a slice of watermelon—is clean and needs no filtration.

Besides the value of the actual *hydration* provided by water, its mineral profile directly influences our health as well. When well hydrated, the body is filled with minerals called electrolytes, which, aptly named, facilitate electrical conduction and communication between neural points. This is how the nervous system sends signals. Inadequate hydration or electrolyte levels can cause faulty communication within the body, producing fatigue, inflammation or sensations of pain, muscle weakness or cramping, dizziness, and even increased chances of illness.[221]

Similarly, the enzymes in our digestive system are hydrolytic, meaning they require water in order to carry out the tasks of digestion. Dehydration can cause us to be unable to properly absorb nutritional intake. This in turn impedes our ability to convert nourishment into energy, effectively store and burn fat, and thus metabolize. As noted earlier, when the metabolic process is impeded, a cycle of other problems begins.

Water also helps detox the body and is vital for regulating temperature—with both processes taking place often through sweat. Likewise, water is the way our system expels toxins and waste through urination and defecation.

For those living in cities, ridding the body of toxins and wastes can be a particular concern, because metropolitan filtration systems often introduce highly toxic chemicals into the water. That's because, first, many public water sources are piped through lead. Second, toxic elements such as chlorine, arsenic, radium, radon, nitrate, fluoride, manganese, uranium, and thorium are often found in municipal water supplies, with some, such as mercury, being detected less often…but it's still possible.[222] Exposure to hazardous chemicals such as these can cause brain damage in children, reproductive issues, nausea, seizures, and an increase in a variety or type of cancer.[223]

Even more frightening for consumers of public water is that it often contains trace amounts of prescription drugs (including antibiotics and even *birth control*) and household chemicals. "In 2008 the U.S. Geological Survey (USGS) tested water in nine states across the country and found that 85 man-made chemicals, including some medications, were commonly slipping through municipal treatment systems and ending up in our tap water."[224] As consumers dispose of these substances, the toxins often find their way into the public waterways, which creates a real filtration problem for the city infrastructure to deal with. The result is that as many as forty-six million Americans have contaminated water flowing into their kitchen and bathroom sinks as they cook and brush their teeth, and cascading across their skin as they shower each day.[225] While many officials claim these numbers are so diminished we shouldn't be worried, we disagree. In fact, experts also concede that they're not sure of precisely *what* risk factors could be "stewing" in our public water supplies, stating that when trace amounts of unknown, various elements are mixed, the results are truly unforeseeable.[226]

Think about this: If you drink water from the tap in the city, you are exposing your body to an unknown array of pharmaceuticals—along with *known* toxins such as arsenic, chloride, and radon—that are likely compromising your health. We strongly suggest that you invest in a water-filtration system and glass water bottles to avoid the BPA (Bisphenol A) and additional toxins carried into your water when stored in plastic), and begin to take your own water when you leave the house. I (Joe) use a Berkey, a gravity-fed water filter that has been proven successful in removing pesticides, herbicides, and other harmful sediments. Just this one change could make a huge difference in your overall health!

Salt

In recent decades, salt has been openly blamed for causing hypertension, cardiovascular and arterial damage, and other imbalances and illness. However, salt is necessary for good health—and it's the white table salt, not sea salt, that deserves censure. Regular white table salt—sodium chloride—is aptly named: sodium and chloride. It has significantly reduced beneficial properties and *can* contribute to health problems. While some of us are taking great pains to eliminate salt from our diets, the truth is, we may need to be salting more— but it's the *type* of salt we need to change, not the amount.

Prepackaged foods are a particular concern; many are over-seasoned with the wrong type of salt. Use caution when purchasing salt advertised as "pink" or "Himalayan," as many imported brands currently on the market are merely regular, iodized salt hiding behind the mask of food dye. On the other hand, healthy salts, such as *real* varieties of pink Himalayan salt or Celtic sea salt, are vital to balance in the body's systems on many levels. They help sustain hydration by providing more than eighty micronutrients such as calcium, potassium, and sodium.[227] Because of their interaction with hydration and electrolytes, they diminish fluid retention and keep muscles hydrated, which lessens muscle cramping.[228] The minerals in sea salts replenish the adrenal glands with necessary sodium and potassium, and fight hypertension while improving skin health with anti-inflammatory agents. The salty taste activates the salivary enzyme amylase and initiates the release of hydrochloric acid within the stomach, helping along the breakdown of nutrition and the metabolizing of calories.[229] I (Joe) start my day with one-fourth of a teaspoon of pink Himalayan salt in about ten ounces of room-temperature water to bolster my adrenals and refresh my lymphatic system. However, we recommend that if you're concerned about increasing your sodium levels, such as those on medications for cardiovascular conditions, consult a natural healthcare practitioner before starting any salt regimen.

Fermented Foods

Probiotics, as mentioned earlier, are bacterial or fungal microorganisms that, "during the fermentation process[,]...convert organic compounds—such as sugars and starch—into alcohol or acids"[230] that serve as preservatives. However, these same agents, when introduced to the body, are known as probiotics, which deliver "good" bacteria to the gut help digestion and nutrient absorption. "Gut flora," as we previously touched on, refers bacteria in the colon. These are vital to our immune system as well as our mental and psychological well-being. They also benefit the rest of our bodies in a number of ways science is even now still discovering. We'll talk more about gut flora in the upcoming pages, but for now we'll cover how eating fermented food benefits this population of small organisms in our intestines.

While there are beneficial bacteria in the gut, there are detrimental ones as well. When the gut has more bad bacteria (small intestinal bacterial overgrowth [SIBO]; Candidas) than good, a condition called dysbiosis sets in. This leads to many digestion issues, such as bloating, constipation, and diarrhea.[231] Thus, keeping the gut balanced is a primary advantage of eating fermented foods via the repopulation of beneficial agents. Additionally, fermented foods are already partially broken down, making the gut's job much easier and causing absorption of nutrients to be simpler for the body. One example of this is phytic acid, which often binds the iron and zinc found in some legumes, making it difficult for the body to take in these minerals. Through fermentation, this factor is diminished and the minerals are available for absorption.[232]

Fermented foods are also beneficial since the secondary exposure to germs on the food help the body build up antibodies. Similar to what we've said regarding local food, when we eat local, organically grown, fermented food loaded with these beneficial organisms, we are exposed to the local bacteria, which helps inoculate against the germs native to our area. Another important aspect of fermentation is found in the fiber itself. When fermented, fiber is in a predigested form, making it very easy on the digestive system. Not only is this fiber a great cleanser, but it is food for bacteria in the gut, providing a good ecological space in which this bacteria can grow. I (Joe) have found that kimchi, raw cheese, sauerkraut, and olives are great fermented foods to work into your diet to keep gut ecology strong.

Gut Health

The value of gut health to our overall wellness is frequently overlooked and underestimated. While we usually recognize the link between the gut and metabolism, many don't know about connections that exist among our brain chemistry, moods, immune system, ability to fight inflammation, and balances in blood sugar, hormones, and other body chemicals. Gut health is covered at more length in *Timebomb*. For additional information on this issue, consider reading that book.

Gut Flora

Gut flora, also known as microbiota, as we've touched on already, break down incoming nutrients and assure that the good ones are properly absorbed and waste is evacuated. The flora are thrown out of balance when we eat processed foods, take antibiotics, or otherwise expose ourselves to chemicals. The constitution of these organisms is vital for more than just digestion. When the colon remains clean, is regularly purged, and isn't continually subjected to damaging food, it remains healthy. When the lining of the gut is compromised, a condition mentioned earlier called leaky-gut syndrome can ensue, which is the beginning of many other chronic illnesses (more on this later). When bacteria are not in balance, additional health risks include cognitive impairments (more on this also, in just a bit), increased inflammation, and gastrointestinal ailments such as Crohn's disease, inflammatory bowel disease (IBD), irritable bowel syndrome (IBS), colitis, diverticular conditions, and many cancers.

Healthy flora helps balance blood sugars, foster emotional and psychological well-being, and increase immunity as well as improve the absorption of nutrients and lower odds of the aforementioned diseases.

In 2018, the American Society for Microbiology published a study that looked at the microbiota of children at age two and compared it with their subsequent BMI (body mass index, a method for measuring body fat) at age twelve. This study selected from children who, at age two, were of similar body mass. The study revealed that while there was no specific indicator that a particular child would one day be obese other than markers found in microbiota, these distinctions existed. It was decided that findings may indicate future propensity toward obesity or an inclination to dietary preferences that would achieve the same result.[233] On this matter, Maggie Stanislawski, medical campus doctor at the University of Colorado Anschutz, stated: "Our study provides more evidence that the gut microbiota might be playing a role in later obesity."[234]

Second Brain

Many recent studies have emerged that refer to the gut as the second brain. Sayings such as "having a gut feeling" or "getting butterflies in the stomach" indicate the link between these two organs.[235] This is based on scientific research regarding something called the enteric nervous system (ENS), which is a system of "100 million nerve cells lining your gastrointestinal tract from esophagus to rectum."[236] This system is responsible for overseeing all digestive processes including, but not limited to, swallowing, releasing digestive enzymes, absorbing nutrients, and eliminating wastes.[237] The ENS is connected to the brain via millions of neurons, keeping the brain greatly in tune with the type of nutrition (or lack thereof) the body is being subjected to. While decades of medical practice have fostered the concept that depression or anxiety leaves us vulnerable to digestive disorders, recent studies have shown the opposite to be true: A poor diet enables emotional instability or mood swings.[238]

In addition, some studies have recently shown a strong correlation between flora imbalances and specific illnesses, meaning that gut bacteria can actually be a predictor of which conditions we may fall prey to. A study using mice showed that those with accelerated negative gut bacteria developed Alzheimer's syndrome through the development of beta-amyloid plaque in the brain.[239] An additional report confirmed a similar result regarding Parkinson's Disease via "alpha-synuclein accumulations and low-grade mucosal inflammation in the enteric nervous system."[240] In other words, imbalance in the gut leads to inflammation, which impacts the brain's cognitive functions.

Timebomb included a lengthy discussion of a wide variety of factors that impact the gut and thus impede the mind. One of the most critical is flora; having the right balance of bacteria is vital. In addition, however, is the matter of processed foods being made with large quantities of flavor enhancers, which are stimulants known as excitotoxins that are able to cross the blood-brain barrier and dramatically affect brain chemistry. These trick the taste buds into believing that the body is having a better food experience than it is in fact having. Further, they biologically addict us to food that is not nutritious. These stimulants have the ability (*as stimulants do*) to cause a constant undertone of anxiety or other psychological upset that we carry throughout the day. (Have you ever eaten junk food, and afterward felt irritable or strangely nervous for no apparent reason?) In this way, our food biologically adds stress to both the gut *and* brain.

An article in *Harvard Health Publishing* states:

A troubled intestine can send signals to the brain, just as a troubled brain can send signals to the gut. Therefore, a person's stomach or intestinal distress can be the cause *or* the product of anxiety, stress, or depression.[241]

As it pertains to the gut's emerging status as the second brain, one thing becomes clear: Creating space in the mind nurtures the digestive tract. However, to achieve this fully, we must also support the intestines so that the mind can be whole.

Immune System

The gut houses 80 percent of the immune system,[242] so is largely responsible for the strength of our immunities many ways. For one thing, as we've emphasized, the gut facilitates the absorption of nutrients, our first defense against illness. Additionally, because of the large quantity of bacteria therein, it is the concentration from which many of our antibodies are born; when flora is out of balance, so is the immune system.[243] When the gut is healthy, we have what we need to fight disease. Unfortunately, many of us are operating with intestines that have vastly compromised health. The symptoms can be so sporadic and seemingly misplaced that they often are allowed to escalate, because we are unaware that our digestive tract's weakness is jeopardizing the condition of the entire body's. When it comes down to it, healthy intestines mean good health, while the adverse means precisely the opposite.

Leaky-Gut Syndrome

A compromised gut is unable to properly break down and process nutrients. When left unaddressed, small openings in the lining of the intestine begin to malfunction, allowing small particles of undigested nutrients to slip into the bloodstream—hence the name leaky-gut syndrome. The liver must then cleanse the particles from the body, causing the alert system to be raised against these substances. This causes a breakdown in the immune system, which results in consequences ranging from food allergies and autoimmune disease to chronic anxiety and depression.

Here's how it works:

———

As the body begins to detect food fragments which have been allowed to escape from a leaking gut, the immune system deploys agents to fight these "enemies." As a result of seeing the need to fight these elements, over time, the body begins to recognize certain foods as being dangerous for the body, thus the development of food allergies. As this issue progresses, the immune system begins to behave erratically as a result of continual overuse and combat triggered by the frequent influx of what it perceives to be intruders (food). Slowly, the immune system reacts in the same way it does when it recognizes an intruder virus or bacteria, which now also burdens the system's filters (the liver, kidneys, etc.) and begins to turn inward, attacking the host, resulting in auto-immune diseases (in which the immune system literally assaults parts of one's own body). As this occurs, the immune system becomes worn out for a few reasons: 1) it's fighting continually, and 2) it cannot be refurbished via incoming nutrition because the gut and immune system are malfunctioning, inhibiting absorption of nutrients, 3) damaged areas cannot properly heal because the body's healing resources are being allocated toward fighting, so the damage to the gut escalates, cutting off the immune system's source of support. Because the body is aware that injury is occurring, it deploys its defense response (which is inflammation) all throughout, causing joints to hurt and sleep to become interrupted and shallow. (In fact, the gut is the greatest inflammation contributor within the entire body). The individual falls into a routine of not getting enough rest and "waking up still tired." Since the immune system is busy (and depleted) fighting its host body, bacterial infections and viruses begin to take hold, causing a person to be continually sick and likely on antibiotics which kill gut flora and perpetuate the problem. Slowly, the body's adrenal resources—which are supposed to be conserved for dangerous situations such as those demanding a fight or flight response—are tapped into more and more regularly as the body seeks resources to continue the combat mode which it is now fully engaged in (against itself) at all times. As adrenal resources are utilized and eventually depleted, illnesses which the body would normally have otherwise been capable of keeping at bay begin to surface, resulting in the need for additional immunal combat and adrenal deployment, which perpetuates the cycle. If this loop isn't interrupted, the individual will eventually become severely chronically ill and this could result in fatality.

———

One of the most important things we can do for our health is avoid falling into this trap. And that's the good news: It's a pitfall we *can* avoid—by eating healthy foods, steering clear of taking gut-destroying antibiotics, and kicking other habits that compromise the lining of the gut. The interesting thing to note about leaky-gut syndrome, as stated before, is that it manifests in many symptoms that, at times, seem unrelated to digestion, such as frequent fatigue or headaches, depression, anxiety, or waves of panic, dehydration, hair loss, insomnia, prediabetes or diabetes, reproductive issues or hormone imbalance, abdominal cramping, liver problems, joint pain, acquired food allergies, kidney problems, heartburn or acid reflux, skin conditions (eczema or acne), autoimmune problems (lupus or Crohn's disease), or bowel issues such as IBD or IBS.

If you suspect you're suffering from leaky-gut syndrome, take heart: It's reversible merely by beginning to take good care of your diet. You can even vastly improve and greatly manage the most severe cases. I (Joe) know this firsthand, as this is the basis of my entire health journey. After two decades of struggling with chronic illness and never having this core issue addressed, I finally began a road to true healing when leaky-gut syndrome was brought to my attention.

Exercise and the Gut

Exercise is a great way to support the gut in its role of digestion. Exercise will be discussed at length in an upcoming chapter, so we'll only briefly touch on the subject here. But, as it pertains to digestion, working out speeds the metabolic process and improves circulation, along with boosting endorphins—which fosters feelings of well-being.[244] When the gut is relaxed, it functions better. In fact, a study released by the University of Gothenburg in 2018 showed that "increased physical activity improves gastrointestinal symptoms in patients with irritable bowel syndrome."[245] On the other hand, numerous studies confirm that a sedentary lifestyle is counter-productive for the bowels.

Herbs and Bitters

Most people are aware of what herbs are, but won't recognize the term "bitters." These are plants that once were used to aid in digestion, but whose use eventually became forgotten or migrated toward distillation for alcoholic purposes; thus, the household recognition and knowledge of them was lost. Herbs and bitters are healthful options that have been forgotten in recent decades, likely out of preference for more palatable foods. That makes perfect sense: In a world filled with delicious, sweet, or savory processed foods or soft drinks loaded with sugars, salts, and flavor enhancers, who wants to take the time or effort to find a source fora dandelion tea or eat an artichoke? Unfortunately, as this thinking has evolved, we've left behind a group of plants that strongly support digestion. Further, foods in this category often aren't subjected to genetic modification as many modern crops have, because their popularity diminished when people started opting for more palatable (often toxic) food choices.[246] Herbs and bitters—some of which are chamomile, burdock, milk thistle, and the aforementioned artichoke and dandelion, just to name a few—yield benefits that include better digestion and nutrient absorption, improved bowel regularity, a suppressed "sweet tooth," anti-inflammatory properties, healthier joints and skin, an elevated mood, and many others.[247] And, because foods such as these haven't been top dietary choices in previous years and have thus escaped the GMO tampering that has befallen so many other plants, they are still extremely nourishing and have even been considered much denser in nutrients than many "superfoods" sold at the grocery stores.[248] Herbs and bitters also soothe and strengthen the body's digestive and detoxification systems.

The Role of Chewing

One of the simplest ways to promote gut health is to thoroughly chew our food. There's no "magic number" of times to do this, because each food has a different consistency. As a general rule, we should chew our food enough so that chunky textures are mashed up well before swallowing.

Chewing food reinforces the digestive process in a few ways. First, the body has a sense of muscle memory that's tied to the act. When the jaw begins working, the lower abdomen begins to relax in preparation for receiving food. (Have you ever eaten in a hurry, and spent the next couple hours feeling as though your midsection was full of rocks?) When these regions relax, the food is processed more slowly and efficiently, which gives the gut an easier time as it processes the nutrients. Fragments of food that aren't chewed can introduce negative bacteria into the gut, throwing off gut flora and leaving us vulnerable to illness.

Additionally, when chewing begins, saliva is dispatched and digestive enzymes are secreted to circulate throughout the throat and stomach, encouraging easier passage of the food through the esophagus. Hydrochloric acid stirs within the stomach to prepare to break down nutrients. These fluids assure that the metabolic process runs smoothly and that digestion occurs in proper timing. When these elements haven't had time to prepare, the result can be bloating, heartburn, indigestion, bowel irregularity, after-meal headache, and fatigue.[249]

Moving Forward

It has been stated in this work, as well as in Joe's previous book, *Timebomb*, that the gut is the epicenter of health for the entire body. Hormonal functions, cognitive processes, immune responses, insulin tolerance, and skeletal, muscular, and vascular health are all affected by what we allow to enter the digestive tract. Yet, for some people, even after addressing such issues as digestive health, there are lingering anomalies in their search for wellness. For these folks, understanding the body's ability to methylate and its need for detox may add a layer of answers and increase their well-being. These topics will be the focus of the next chapter.

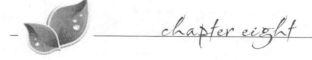

chapter eight

Methylation, MTHFR, and Detoxification

Methylation. You may not be familiar with that term, and even if you are, you may find it intimidating. However, since methylation affects all aspects of our health, it's important to address it. The reader may recognize the word, but find themselves wondering what it means. A quick Google search of the term has great potential to worsen a person's confusion on the subject. Worse, it seems that nearly daily the media is filled with new and even conflicting data, which seems to be currently emerging at a rapid pace. While a thorough study of this process could easily be (and *is*) the topic of many books, we'll do our best to keep the complicated topic as simple and palatable as possible. The first step, then, is a definition.

What Is Methylation?

The term "methylation" refers to a process that takes place at the cellular level throughout the entire body. Since the body functions using proteins such as hormones and enzymes (just to name a couple), cells attach what is known as "methyl groups…a chemical structure made of one carbon and three hydrogen atoms"[250] to these molecules in order to control how the body responds to them, thus defining (and sometimes altering) the benefits or drawbacks derived from anything taken in to the body. This can refer to food ingested, chemicals breathed, or even substances applied topically. This process is known as methylation. When the body can methylate properly, nutrients are taken in and absorbed as they should be, but when the body is unable to properly undergo this process, health problems can be the result.[251] While many elements can hinder the body's ability to methylate properly, one emergent area of recognition and concern is genetic MTHFR variants.

What Is MTHFR?

MTHFR is an abbreviation for methylenetetrahydrofolate reductase, an enzyme involved in the body's methylation cycle. It should be noted before moving on that there is a MTHFR *gene* that writes the code into the agent it sends into the body: the MTHFR *enzyme*. Many mistakenly believe that the determination of good or bad methylation is made by the enzymatic agents working within the body—but that's only partially the case. The *true* key to successful methylation is when the gene that codes these agents programs them successfully. However, for some, the MTHFR gene itself has a deviation that causes it to poorly encrypt the enzyme it sends out. When this happens, methylation can quickly become more challenging.

Methylation and Nutrient Absorption

For those who have an MTHFR variant or other methylating issue, the body has problems properly absorbing nutrients and expelling toxins. The resulting nourishment deficiencies or stacked pollutants found within the body then potentially set the stage for illness to occur. For example, homocysteine is a common but toxic amino acid found in the blood of many of us, often as a result of eating meat. Through methylation, the body is *usually* able to convert this substance into its beneficial counterpart: methionine. How does this change take place? As it pertains to homocysteine, the MTHFR enzyme plays a large role in the body's detoxification process via a chain reaction which involves the cofactor 5,10-methylenetetrahydrofolate becoming 5-methyltetrahydrofolate, which then creates methionine from homocysteine utilizing an enzyme called methionine synthase.[252]

Complicated—right? In English: The MTHFR enzyme operates to ensure that several complicated chemical conversions take place so that the body absorbs every nutrient it possibly can, and that the rest is flushed from the system without incident. So, when the MTHFR gene properly codes the enzyme, methylation is successful. When the MTHFR gene is deviated (or other communicational pathways in the body inhibit methylation), it is unable to properly encrypt its agent, and methylation fails.

This is where pointing out methylation as a contributing culprit to other illness becomes vague. After all, the nutshell definition of methylation is the body's ability to discern the nature of all incoming elements—both toxic and nutritious—and then absorb or dispose of them accordingly. How, then, can poor methylation lead to advanced health issues? Consider the already mentioned example of homocysteine. It has been stated that this is a common element in many people's systems. It is brought in via meat (which *should* boost our protein nutrients)—so it would appear harmless, or even healthy, right? However, homocysteine, unchecked, has been linked to heart disease, stroke, dementia, hypertension, vascular issues, hypothyroidism, diabetes, high cholesterol, and other complications. This situation becomes a key identifier in showing how the level at which an individual methylates can be a vital marker in overall health. As is with the case of homocysteine, optimum methylation is necessary for the conversion from a negative protein to a beneficial one to take place within the body, otherwise toxins remain rampant in the bloodstream, leaving us vulnerable to disease.[253] This is only one type of substance that can mount up in the system as a result of poor methylation. Other toxins left unchecked can lead to complications that include but aren't limited to vitamin and mineral deficiency; neurotransmitter communication that can contribute to anxiety, bipolar disorder, and schizophrenia;[254] and depression, autism, and migraines.[255] Because functional, healthy detoxification is so important to cellular health, advanced methylation impediment can indirectly contribute to many forms of cancer such as colon cancer and leukemia[256] and can be the underlying culprit for inflammation, chronic pain, nerve pain, fatigue, and obesity.[257] On an even more somber note, this issue can cause reproductive problems, birth defects, and miscarriages as well.[258] For many women who have repeatedly had trouble conceiving or carrying a pregnancy to full term may unknowingly have an MTHFR deviation or another methylating challenge as the source of their issue.

Does This Even Apply To Me?

At this point, you might be thinking, "I don't have a diagnosis of inhibited methylation such as an MTHFR variant. So, this scenario doesn't apply to me." Allow us to challenge this thinking by pointing out that many doctors agree that, for a mixture of reasons—some of which are genetic, while others are environmental—between 40 to 60 percent of the population doesn't methylate properly. Recall the example already given of impeded methylation of homocysteine potentially contributing to such issues as heart disease, stroke, dementia, hypertension, vascular issues, hypothyroidism, diabetes, and even conditions as seemingly ordinary as high cholesterol. For this reason, keep an open mind as you take in the information in the upcoming pages. As we'll delve into momentarily, a diagnosis of a named condition such as MTHFR isn't not the only culprit which may mean that the body doesn't methylate properly. Perhaps a missing link in your search for wellness is about to be revealed.

Furthermore, proper/improper methylation has the potential to alter how our bodies function all the way down to the cellular-genetic level. Since our genes are also proteins, methylation has the potential to alter gene expression: meaning genes can literally be switched on or off depending on how the process is working in an individual's body. This has the power to steer health in a positive or negative direction, which is why knowledge regarding whether your body is successfully completing this process is critical to good health.

Before Latching On to a Treatment Plan

For many, a quick research on improved methylation yields myriad suggestions to supplement with B-complex vitamins, asserting these supplements as though they were a "one size fits all" answer to such issues. Others often endorse folate or methylfolate. However, before readers race to purchase these supplements, they should be aware that there could be a few problems with this approach. First, quality and absorbability of such products is vital: if you have an obstacle with methylation, it may be even harder for you to absorb certain supplements than it is for most other people. Thus, high-quality supplements are necessary. Additionally, there are different types of MTHFR mutations/variants and other methylation impediments, and these issues aren't all the same. It may surprise you to learn this, but there are people who don't methylate properly who likewise *do not* have a condition—genetic or otherwise—that doctors might "flag" as responsible for their methylation struggles. What we mean is that some who have a methylation issue battle with symptoms derived from an ambiguous source, but repeatedly may be told by physicians that they're unable to find a diagnosable problem. (These same people may even test negative for all MTHFR variants). This is because the matter is extremely complex and can be derived not only from genetic factors (which may be diagnosable), but from environmental ones as well (which often do not show up on a diagnostic test of any kind).

To elaborate, the human genome contains between four to five million SNPs (single nucleotide polymorphisms). These can each cause unique variations in an individual's base genetic makeup. They contribute to all of the various elements which make each of us unique in every way, and furthermore, "act as biological markers, helping scientists locate genes that are associated with disease. When SNPs occur within a gene or in a regulatory region near a gene, they may play a more direct role in disease by affecting the gene's function."[259] But the issue of methylation goes beyond our genetics—and is thus not limited by them (thankfully!). A person's ability to methylate, as staged in part by our genetic pattern at birth, is subsequently influenced by literally millions of decisions we make throughout our lives. This involves every exposure we allow our bodies to withstand over the course of our existence, from pollutants and food ingredients to topical chemical exposure, and can even include some vaccines.

With this in mind, it goes without saying that it's impossible (nor is it reasonable for us to expect) for a medical professional to have both the foreknowledge of the intricacies of each patient's genetic patterns, along with the ability to calculate and comprehend the consequences of each of our decisions across our lifetimes and how each of these factors intertwines to impact our health. Even the best professionals find themselves unable to provide unlimited expertise regarding such vast and unknowable circumstances and influencing factors. The mere fact that methylation can be impacted over decades of our lives via the choices that we make, by genetic variations inherited from our parents, or both, means that the roots of methylation problems can be ambiguous to trace. What we're saying is that it isn't as simple as "getting tested" for a named condition such as MTHFR, and then working purely from a genetic standpoint to resolve. Likewise, doing a quick Google search and then adding touted supplements will likely not manifest a simple answer to the problem. As stated previously, those who test negative for such conditions may still have impeded methylation due to blocked pathways (more on pathways in a bit) in their system as a result of poor diet, pollutant or chemical exposure, or other life decisions that have compromised the body's ability to methylate.

There Is Good News

Before continuing, we want to take a moment to reemphasize how important all the principles in this book are for a healthy lifestyle that follows natural protocol. By embracing a way of life based on these methods, we provide our bodies with many of the best tools available for improved methylation. Unfortunately, sometimes the search to "overcome MTHFR" or "repair a methylation dysfunction" becomes the entire focus of the journey, and the fixation is skewed from seeking out the healthiest lifestyle possible to one of fighting a battle against genetics. This is a discouraging war, and should be avoided by committing to offer our bodies every opportunity to thrive naturally.

Since methylation is a highly personalized issue, many times another individual's claim of having found the "magic, silver bullet" that effectively treated his or her MTHFR/methylation issue will result in the well-meaning comrade sharing their suggestions of treatment and tales of victory that do not render the same results for another person. This can become a spiral of defeat for the individual still searching for his or her optimum treatment blend, and this is a distraction from the *real* journey we should be on: that of arming our body with the best tools it needs to thrive, and then allowing it time to heal. The habits suggested throughout this book—especially for the individual with methylation difficulty—will help your body adapt to a lifestyle in which is it able to detox safely and organically, thus facilitating the eventuality of improved methylation and function on many levels.

Pathways

We have mentioned pathways before, and at this point the reader may be wondering what is meant by this. Pathways are the totality of the body's various types of internal communication systems. They include (but aren't limited to) the metabolic, neurological, endocrine, and nervous systems. "These systems regulate body processes through chemical and electrical signals that pass between cells. The pathways for this communication are different for each system."[260] For example, "the nervous and endocrine systems are two forms of communication system in the human body that integrate, coordinate and respond to sensory information which is received by the human body from its surroundings"[261] (i.e. diet, stressors, lifestyle, pesticides, herbicides, heavy metals, parasites, environmental, etc.). This means that when these communications are inhibited, vital body functions such as the intake and absorption of nutrients, hormone production, ability to sleep, energy production, and the ability to methylate properly become dysfunctional. Many Americans, whether they know it or not, face the types of toxins mentioned previously that block or derange their pathways (which should be open).

Because improper methylation can result in the body's inability to intake nutrients, the issue is often initially detected via nutritional deficiency. Understandably, the response is usually to add the deprived nutrient to the system through supplementation. Many individuals who have been diagnosed with MTHFR or other methylating disorder immediately begin a myriad of supplementation to try to improve methylation. But this can prove to have devastating side effects, because it can result in an individual's already-strained metabolic pathways becoming overloaded and thus locked. What this means is that adding supplementation to a deficiency is not *always* the answer. Until the issue of impeded pathways is addressed, taking supplements will likely only exacerbate the problem. In this type of situation, the body will "clog" with these elements, putting undue strain on liver and kidneys, while the individual simultaneously remains unable to absorb them at all.

I (Joe) experienced this when I first learned that I had two genetic Methylenetetrahydrofolate reductase (MTHFR) variations/mutations (heterozygous and homeozygus, 677T and A1298C) and began taking methyl-B complexes, because further testing confirmed I had become enormously vitamin B deficient. Initially I felt relief, but then as these substances mounted in my body unabsorbed, my system became so completely overloaded that I began to feel terribly sick, as though I had toxins all throughout my body despite my carefully regimented organic diet. And this was the case: the over-supplementation had stacked in my system, because my body could not methylate (break down, absorb, use, and store these nutrients) resulting in a stockpile of partially-methylated nutrients which became a burden of additional waste on my body. This created neurotoxins, which brought about feelings of illness, chills, and even brain fog that seemed impossible to work through. At a later time, I had a similar issue regarding iron: I was deficient (borderline anemic), and yet simultaneously, my blood held large stores of this micronutrient (in the form of ferritin), seemingly unabsorbable (more on this in just a bit).

This is where the situation with treating MTHFR or other methylation issues becomes complicated. There are many great natural healthcare practitioners out there who are able to help, but there is, unfortunately, no "cookie cutter" treatment which is proven to alleviate issues for everybody, or for every case. Because the MTHFR variant occurs within the genetic code, management of this condition becomes highly personalized to each individual. Additionally, as stated, many will be quick to subscribe to a wide regimen of supplementation in effort to balance nutrients which appear deficient. Allow me to say that for an individual with a methylation imbalance, this can be a serious mistake before peripheral issues, such as pathways, have been addressed.

Cofactors, Precursors, and Methyl Mountain

When I first discovered I had MTHFR variants, I aggressively began to purchase supplements and follow protocols of choline, methyl folate, glutathione, vitamins A and E, and fish oil—and, for a time, I felt amazing. After years of struggling with illness, imagine my thrill at getting some relief! I felt better than I had in years; it was as though I had a new lease on life. This "high," which I later called "methyl mountain," lasted for a few months. Then, to my *unspeakable* dismay, my symptoms returned. At the time, I was crushed: I was disappointed that the discomfort had reemerged, afraid that it had returned to stay, and unsure of what I had done wrong since, I had been so rigid about my new wellness routine that had *previously* been working.

However, I soon learned that the intricacies of nutrient intake can be extremely complicated for an individual facing methylation challenges. Likewise, many people fail to realize that nutrients have cofactors and precursors that are required in order to allow absorption to successfully take place. Bear with me while I attempt to explain this.

You may have heard it said that calcium cannot be absorbed unless a person takes it along with vitamin D. In fact, many vitamin companies have capitalized on this commonly known fact by packaging and advertising the two together for purposes of better absorption. This is because vitamin D facilitates the gut's ability to intake calcium, after which it is vitamin K which actually helps direct the calcium to the bones. Many people regard nutrients as separate, stand-alone entities that move through the body independently and do their job, but this is mistaken. Each essential element belongs to a chain-link of necessary components the body needs *in succession* in order to thrive. Likewise, each has precursors and cofactors that facilitate their impact upon the body.

As in my aforementioned case regarding coexistent ferritin and anemia, because I had stores of excess iron in my body that had been unabsorbed, taking more iron (to help my anemia) would have caused more illness, because my body already had enough in storage (ferritin). It's not that I didn't have any; it was that my body was unable to absorb it properly. In my case, chlorophyll and vitamin C, along with exercise and lots of sunshine (vitamin D and oxygenation) would prove far more effective cofactors for helping my body to actually utilize the iron that was already present, pulling it out of storage and into circulation. (Chlorophyll is a green pigment, present in all green plants and in cyanobacteria, responsible for the absorption of light to provide energy for photosynthesis. And interestingly, vitamin C assists in the efficiency of glutathione by up to 30 percent, which is a vital antioxidant that also helps with methylation.) What is needed in such situations is to decipher which cofactor or precursor is needed to get the body to absorb what is already there.

In addition, sometimes we may think we need a certain nutrient, and, after beginning to take it, we find that we feel much better—for a while. Unfortunately, this can be followed by the grandiose letdown when symptoms return (as did following my brief visit to "methyl mountain"). It's easy in such circumstances to feel extremely defeated, having had a taste of relief that is followed by recurring discomfort. In such cases, it's likely that when we first initiate supplementation, we have a supply of the right cofactor or precursor in our system, which facilitates absorption of the supplement. However, this element will likely deplete as it aids in the absorption of the *known*, culprit deficiency. As we continue taking this essential, we are unaware that intake has been aided by another component until the second, *assisting* essential similarly becomes depleted. Then, as a result of lack of appropriate cofactor, the body begins to struggle at intake of the item being supplemented, which allows for the return of initial symptoms. The result, in such situations, is often the discouragement of experiencing diminished success in spite of faithful efforts. I know this feeling all too well, the cruel tease of what was almost obtained, then lost without explanation.

The Big Picture—It All Works Together

When we don't consider pathways, cofactors, and precursors, it can be extremely discouraging. As I've related, I (Joe) have experienced first-hand the cycle of supplementing in an attempt to fill a deficiency and feeling better for a while, just to have hopes come crashing down again as discomfort and symptoms return. This is both a physical and an emotional roller-coaster ride that comes from being unable to pinpoint the deficiency what cofactors or precursors help absorption. Sometimes it takes persistence and further investigation to get to the heart of the issue; we must know our deficiencies *as well as* the influencing assistance of other factors that aid the intake of these elements. Additionally, before supplementation can be successful, we must make sure that pathways aren't blockaded in order for the body to even be able to accept the nutrients. You may be wondering *how* your pathways can be cleaned. One powerful method of opening up the body's pathways is to implement a systematic approach to detoxification (the removal of heavy metals, pesticides, toxic chemicals, and other environmental pollutants that disrupt the body's regulatory and communication systems; more on detox in a bit). Beyond this, none of these measures will be completely successful until the principles in this book have been implemented and followed as a lifestyle.

In addition, I (Joe) often recommend a strategic detox for most individuals *long before* I suggest they start consuming a new supplement or nutrient. Detox is a regimen that actually begins by cleaning up our diet and adding lifestyle changes such as increased sun exposure and quality sleep. Detoxing the body's communication pathways prepares the body to receive nutrition, and can help minimize nutrient-overload.

No Cookie-Cutter Regimen

Often, we view natural healthcare practitioners as experts at dealing with each case of MTHFR or methylation impediment. However, the fact that this issue can be impacted by everything from genetic makeup to what we eat and put on our skin makes it far too ambiguous for these professionals to effectively trace and pinpoint. They have a limited amount of knowledge about us (the extent of that knowledge is literally confined to the information exchanged during office visits), while they're being asked to share with us their expertise regarding the most complicated, vague, and anomalous questions concerning our health. Likewise, the seeker is often looking for that "magic, silver bullet" supplement or that "cookie-cutter" regimen that has been proven to reverse symptoms and "solve the problem." While many devoted individuals in this field are qualified and capable, the personalized nature of MTHFR variants and other methylation issues and their need for exclusively tailored treatments can mean that the path to relief requires open communication, patience, persistence, and the understanding that there's no one-size-fits-all method for treatment.

Please know that I truly understand that putting all of this together and allowing time for the body to respond—while searching out cofactors and precursors in conjunction with trying to unblock pathways—can seem overwhelming. At times, when you experience a downward tick (such as my descent from methyl mountain), you may feel defeated and financially deflated, having put many resources into the wrong (often costly) supplements. I urge you to keep an open mind, and try not to become discouraged. During moments like this, those who become frustrated may be tempted to believe that the natural path is both expensive and ineffective. This isn't the case, but you need to fully understand that successful treatment may take time, persistence, patience, and even some trial and error until you can dial in on the right strategy.

Natural Life: The First Step

It bears repeating that the wellness techniques presented in this book are the first step you can take toward good health, and this is true for proper methylation as well. These principles have secured a more consistent and sustainable health for me (Joe) than any other methodology available. I get my vitamin D from sunshine, my choline and vitamin B-12 from farm-fresh eggs, and my riboflavin (B-2) from dark, leafy greens. I've never enjoyed long-lasting wellness that compares to the quality of life I currently maintain, and it's because the way God created our bodies to interact with His creation was done with purpose, intention, and abundant provision. However, it was intended to be followed as a *lifestyle*. Supplements are wonderful, but we can't "supplement" our way out of a sedentary way of life, a reckless diet, or sleep deprivation. We have to prioritize our health, then follow the protocol each day—regardless of whether it is convenient (this is especially true for those with MTHFR variant or other methylation issue). We simply *must* commit to guard our wellness and see it through.

If You Really Want to Know

If you feel that information on your genetics may give you insight on your health, and you want to obtain a genetic test for MTHFR deviations or other genetic variables, they are available through medical doctors, many natural healthcare practitioners, and even online. If you find that you have one of these mutations, we cannot stress to you enough the importance of understanding that *this does not equate to a future diagnosis of disease*. Remember that environmental culprits can impact methylation as well as genetics, and genetics can adapt to operate differently, depending on your decisions. Thus, you're not limited to, nor are you equivalent to, the numbers that show in your genetic code. After all, a those diagnosed with an MTHFR variant may develop a heightened vigilance with which they guard their health with every precaution, ultimately resulting in better overall health than others who may have had no genetic predisposition to poor methylation, but who took no precautions regarding their health. Thus, our proactive lifestyle choices can contribute more to our overall well-being than our genetic code.

However, a diagnosis of an issue such as an MTHFR variant can alert us to the fact that we, potentially more than most people, need to be very careful about following the principles outlined in this book. Knowing about a condition such as MTHFR variant will also let us know that our body (if left unaided) may have more trouble absorbing vitamin and mineral supplements than the average person, and merely adding deficient nutrients may not solve the problem. For those with methylation issues, it is extra-important to take in vitamins and minerals in conjunction with precursors and cofactors, and to take in these elements through diet as often as possible. Also, because the detox process may present additional challenges, it is imperative to be extremely cautious regarding what we put into our bodies in the first place, *especially* for those with a diagnosed methylation disorder. Healthy, organic food, free of chemicals, dyes, flavor enhancers, or other toxins are vital for future health. Make a resolution to avoid simple carbs, toxic ingredients, and processed or prepackaged foods. Additionally, avoid harsh household or commercial chemicals, paint fumes, heavy perfumes, or topical hygienic products such as deodorant containing aluminum, which the body has a difficult time ridding itself of. We can't emphasize enough how important it is, in today's world (filled with pollutants, toxic food ingredients, and other exposing elements), for *everyone* to take intentional strides toward detoxing their systems, but this is particularly true for people who are struggling with methylation difficulties.

MTHFR: Not The Cause or the Illness

While MTHFR isn't considered the underlying *cause* of chronic illness, it is gaining recognition by many doctors as contributing to the body's inability to overcome certain difficulties. Also, 50 percent of the American population and 95 percent of autistic or spectrum disorder patients show evidence of MTHFR variation.[262] It is possible that you've been on a vague, ill-defined quest for answers to ambiguous health issues. If this is the case, it could be that poor methylation (such as MTHFR or similar condition) has contributed to your anomalous health issues. For many, uncovering this key ingredient in their own cycle toward wellness has opened doors for treatment and healing that would have otherwise been closed. However, many struggle with methylation unaware and fail to realize that the correlating symptoms can be as subtle as folate and B deficiency, fatigue, shortness of breath, constipation, loss of appetite or unintentional weight loss, muscle weakness, numbness, tingling, or pain in the hands or feet, dizziness or loss of balance, mouth sores, mood changes, or anemia (which may manifest signs of fatigue, weakness, shortness of breath, dizziness, or irregular heartbeat, and for which a person should consult a doctor).

Other Steps

It has been well emphasized at this point that the principles in this book will help you develop a healthy lifestyle which, on its own, will likely improve your methylation and natural well-being. However, there are additional steps you can take to alleviate the physical challenges that come along with MTHFR and other methylation problems. Here are a few suggestions:

1. Remove *all* grains, alcohol, sugar, and processed foods from your diet immediately.
2. Avoid environmental toxins such as artificially scented air fresheners and non-natural cleaning chemicals.
3. Switch to natural skin and hair products (this includes lotions, toothpaste, and deodorant).
4. Exercise to detox—if you are physically able. Make sure you work up a good sweat! (Infrared saunas can help as well.)

5. Get more sleep, and better-quality sleep.

6. Increase greens and cruciferous veggies—an important source of B vitamins!

7. Talk to your natural healthcare practitioner about taking methylated folate (vitamin B-9), methylcobalamin (B-12), betaine in the form of TMG, NAC, glutathione, pyridoxal-5-phosphate (vitamin B-6), riboflavin, (vitamin B-2), and curcumin.

8. Decrease stress, and spend time in prayer and meditation regarding the good things God has done for you.

9. Eat fermented foods (as mentioned previously).

10. Take regular detox baths (discussed in upcoming pages).

11. Limit exposure to wi-fi technology and avoid activities that require prolonged digital screen time.

12. PLEASE NOTE: A small number of people with MTHFR (if you can imagine) actually *over*-methylate! They are unable to tolerate methylated products well, if at all. Therefore, folic acid *and* methylfolate, methylcobalamine, etc. (often presumed to be the go-to regimen for those starting treatment for MTHFR), will make their symptoms worse. (I [Joe] believe, at least in part, this is one of the reasons for the challenges I've experienced.)

Detox

Because of the burden placed on the body's sensory and communication pathways by today's environmental pollutants, toxic food ingredients, topical chemical compounds, and other elements we're exposed to daily, detoxification is one of the most important things we can do for our health. Detox is not a one-time event, it's part of a lifestyle that we must discover and follow faithfully, *each and every day*. When considering detox, keep the following three points in mind:

1. There is no one-size-fits-all method for detoxing; everyone's body is different.

2. As mentioned previously, when we live by the principles endorsed in this book, we organically dwell in a detoxifying lifestyle. Thus, before subscribing to any detox regimen, implement these habits and allow your body time to adapt to them before adding an actual detox method or any additional supplements/protocols. (In this way, *this* book is the guide for a healthy, safe, long-term detoxification plan for your body.)

3. Possibly most importantly: Understand that any additional measure you take to attempt detox should be done with the help of a natural healthcare practitioner. Detoxing can be dangerous if the method you choose is too fast or too severe, because it demands a lot from the body. I (Joe) once did a detox procedure too quickly and used measures that were too extreme, and became *terribly* nauseous for six weeks. I later learned that when we do this, the body can go into mild shock, and the symptoms can include bowel disruption, stomach cramps, gas and bloating, headaches, skin irritation, fatigue, mood swings, cravings, restlessness, insomnia, sinus congestion, low-grade fever, cold or flu-like symptoms, and anxiety. Additionally, we may have secondary elements inhibiting the body's ability to detox—such as the possibility of a parasite—which may require the help of a natural healthcare practitioner for identification and treatment. (Parasites, while outside the scope of this book, can be the culprits or contributing factors to anomalous and recurring health issues. For those suffering with persistent health troubles, it may be beneficial to address this possibility with the assistance of a natural healthcare practitioner.)

4. The liver plays a vital role in detox by processing and packaging unwanted toxins (pesticides, herbicides, heavy metals, etc.) for removal from the body. However, once prepared, they still

need to be physically expelled from your body—either through defecation, urination, breathing, or sweating. As discussed earlier, the gut also plays an *enormous* part in the daily detox processes. This, in part, is why we have placed so much emphasis on gut health throughout this book. Our gut flora must be healthy and balanced with the correct bacterial makeup, and it's vital that it be able to mobilize the hefty number of toxic waste products that the liver is preparing for removal. So, if the digestive system isn't balanced during the detox process, many harsh toxins can accumulate in the bloodstream, as well as tissues placing the brain and body under unsustainable toxic loads. Excess toxicity such as this becomes difficult to secrete through normal detox pathways (urination, defecation, sweat, etc.). Thus, they begin looking for another escape route—via the skin, the lungs, and/or the kidneys. The result can include a number of detrimental detox symptoms, such as acne; bumpy, itchy or sensitive skin; rashes; eczema (atopic dermatitis); hives; pronounced body odor; strong-smelling sweat; bad breath; headaches; brain fog; or darkly colored urine.

Ask Your Natural Healthcare Practitioner Before Taking These Natural Detox Aids

We've already stated that you should consider the principles in this book to be a great way to begin the detox process (getting daily doses of sunlight, regular exercise, sweating, getting quality sleep, eating "clean," taking in fresh air, etc.). We've likewise emphasized that we believe it's ill-advised to consult the Internet for radical methods regarding extreme detox pertaining to heavy metals, pesticides, and other environmental toxins, and then immediately jump into such programs on the first day. Advanced detox should be undertaken slowly, carefully, and after enlisting the help of a trained professional. However, for the sake of information, we want to share a list of additional points to consider using *at the advice of a natural healthcare practitioner.* Many products on the market claim to cleanse, detox, purify, or otherwise remove unwanted substances from the body, but many are either ineffective or are made of harsh chemicals. To educate the reader on the matter of understanding what is available to them and to render a quick understanding of terminology, we offer here a list of *all-natural* substances that will likely be suggested by your natural healthcare practitioner. Once you've been given the green light from a professional regarding what's listed here, you'll likely find many of these are useful.

Milk Thistle: Often referred to as the "King Herb" for liver detox, this contains the active ingredient silymarin, which acts as an antioxidant by reducing free radical production and creates a detoxifying effect. This is why milk thistle has been linked to a multitude of benefits regarding liver support and overall detox.

Glutathione: Known as the "Mother of all Antioxidants," this is one of the most powerful endogenous antioxidants in the entire body. It's extremely powerful anti-inflammatory, detoxification, and neuroprotective abilities help prevent aging, cancer, heart disease, dementia, and more. Doctors have used glutathione to treat everything from autism to Alzheimer's disease.

L-glutamine: Glutamine is an amino acid used in the biosynthesis of proteins. Its side chain is similar to that of glutamic acid, except the carboxylic acid group is replaced by an amide. It is known to help heal leaky-gut syndrome as well as enhance liver detoxification.

B-Complex: B vitamins play a major role in running the first phase of liver detoxification, especially vitamins B2, B3, B6, folate, and B12.

Alginate from seaweed: Sodium alginate is enormously effective at binding with heavy metals in the gut and bloodstream for safe elimination from the body. It also provides great support to your body's detoxification processes.

Selenium: (Se) This has been shown to counteract the dangerous toxicity of heavy metals including cadmium, methylmercury, inorganic mercury, thallium, and to a limited extent, silver.

Zinc: Zinc is a strong antioxidant that helps destroy and eliminate free radicals, as well as assists in removing heavy metals from the body.

Vitamin C: Vitamin C flushes (ascorbate cleanses) are prescribed by many doctors to help rid the body of innumerable toxins. The typical method is to introduce high dietary amounts of vitamin C until a watery stool is produced. Vitamin C helps eliminate dangerous free radicals from the body as well.

N-acetylcysteine: NAC is a potent amino acid that helps increase glutathione levels, which helps protect the liver and kidneys from toxic injury. It is also known to aid in maintaining good pulmonary health due to its mucolytic activity.

Alpha-lipoic acid: Supports liver detoxification and has powerful antioxidant effects that greatly support nerve health and mental sharpness.

Detox Teas

In addition to lifestyle changes and professionally guided detox supplementation, many teas can be beneficial in ridding the body of toxins. Some of the benefits associated with the detoxifying herbal teas listed below include reducing belly bloat, relieving stress and anxiety, improving immunity, relieving constipation, cleansing the liver and colon, lowering inflammation, facilitating weight loss, relieving cramps, stimulating brain function, treating indigestion, regulating blood-sugar levels, soothing intestinal walls, helping to treat infections, eliminating toxins, and even improving the health of the skin.

Indian sarsaparilla root: Traditionally known for its use in flavoring root beer, people have also used sarsaparilla for centuries as a tonic because of its detoxifying properties.

Ginger root: In ayurvedic (alternative medicine, often referring to ancient Eastern) medicine, ginger is incredibly useful, and is also used to treat a variety of conditions, including discomfort related to the digestive tract.

Burdock root: This is a member of the daisy family, and can be a phenomenal way to help cleanse the liver.

Black pepper: Pepper contains piperine, which helps prevent fat cell differentiation, increases the bio-availability (absorbtion) of nutrients, and is full of antioxidants.

Dandelion root: The dandelion plant (both the root and leaf) is, as mentioned previously, known as a "bitter" and holds all the health benefits associated with this category of herbs. These offer assistance priming the digestive system for optimal function, and are an effective detoxifying agent for the kidneys and liver.

Juniper berry extract: This might be best known for its use as a flavoring in European cuisine, but it also helps support kidney function, cleanses the urinary tract, and relieves intestinal gas.

Detox Diet

As stated previously, we should always try to eat healthy, organic food free of toxic ingredients, but certain foods foster detoxification. Making the intentional effort to add the following foods the the diet yields vast detoxification advantages: cilantro, garlic, wild blueberries, lemon water, spirulina, chlorella, barley grass juice powder, atlantic dulse, and garlic (just to name a few).

Detox Baths

One additional method of cleansing the body of toxins is detox baths, for which there are many techniques and recipes. We've stressed the importance of good exercise, which gives the body the opportunity to expel toxins from the body via sweat. Similarly, it has been mentioned that the skin is the body's largest organ, so a hot bath can be a relaxing way to reward yourself for putting in a good workout. Detox baths, filled with the correct balance of natural, safe ingredients—such as Epsom salt (magnesium sulfate), ginger, and essentials oils such as lavender and lemon—soothe muscles and joints, draw out toxins, and fortify the body with vital minerals and nutrients.

Choices

As we've done so often in the book to this point, we want to take a moment to reassure you that if you've experienced symptoms discussed in this chapter, be encouraged. Many people who have made mistakes with their bodies have continued, after adopting health-fostering habits, to live long and happy, healthy lives.

Most who acquire health problems from eating toxic food or being exposed to dangerous chemical compounds made those unwise decisions in ignorance. However, just as God showed me (Daniel) the need to wade into fresh water even when I didn't understand the scientific reason for why it would help my body, abiding in God's laws teaches us what we need to know when we submit to His will and commit to live in the ways He directs.

We've already stated that the choices we make literally have the power to change our bodies on a genetic level. But recall the first and most important thing about us as human beings, as told to us in Genesis 1:27: We're made in the image of God.

This means that our Creator loves us and wants to restore us. No power on earth can keep us from His love (Romans 8:38–39). Ultimately, the God who loves us will bless the efforts we make when we surrender to His will.

Does this mean all will experience miraculous healing in this lifetime? We wish we could say the answer is yes, but that simply wouldn't be true. However, we've discussed what true healing has been provided by Jesus' stripes, and nothing can take this from His children. God is always extending help to those who ask for it, and as we continue our journey toward pursuing what is good, He will extend us grace.

chapter nine

Exercise and Activity

Everybody these days seems to know that exercise is critical to good health. Most people are aware that it burns excess calories and fights obesity. They also know on some level that exercise gets the blood pumping, so is connected to cardiovascular health. Beyond these principles, many don't understand the extent to which exercise is critical to overall good health: Every system in the body benefits from exercise, including the brain, the circulatory system, heart, lungs, liver, metabolism, and even the immune system.[263]

Unfortunately, knowing that we *should* exercise regularly and actually doing it are two very different things. The CDC has recognized that 80 percent of Americans don't get enough activity to sustain good health.[264]

At this time, the conversation often migrates toward resources such as gym memberships, fitness apps, or (expensive) personal trainers. However, just as quickly as we decide to entertain such thoughts, we usually dismiss them. Where gyms are concerned, we seem to lack the follow-through it takes to visit more than a couple times before the only memory of the new workout plan is the debited funds drawn unrewarded from our checking account in subsequent months. Statistics show that there is an average spike, peaking as much as 34–50 percent higher than usual, on January 1 of nearly any given year, but by the third

Thursday of January of the same year, a decline begins that lasts until about the first of March, whereupon user numbers usually diminish to the previous year's averages.[265]

There are many reasons we don't follow through after joining a gym, including, but not limited to, various forms of body shaming, which makes weight loss or visible results, rather than quality of life, the motivation for exercise.[266] Think about the way most of us tend to play comparison games while working out. We may feel awkward using equipment in front of others whose bodies are more fit; we may be embarrassed about not knowing how equipment operates; we might be uncomfortable undressing in the locker rooms; or we might even dread the part that has us sweating and panting in a room filled with strangers. These are all understandable concerns, and they don't even reflect those who don't join a gym in the first place because the expense, scheduling demands, or inconvenient location is prohibitive. As a result, many of us don't think we have the availability or power to take charge of our health in this way.

However, outspoken advocates for exercise explain that "promoting exercise for physical appearance further idealizes thinness and further exacerbates weight stigma... [but] when we start exercising for pleasure and fun, exercise can become intrinsically motivating, meaning we are motivated from within."[267]

This means that when we remove our focus from the concept that workouts should take place a set number of times per week at a set location, and for a set amount of time, we can get a liberating new perspective on exercise. Instead of forcing a cumbersome workout regimen into our already-busy lives, we should—as discussed in a previous chapter—begin by creating space. Once our schedules allow some time for leisure, then we can think about what types of physical activity we would *also* consider fun.

There's a novel notion, right?

This could mean that we exercise by gardening, swimming, dancing, or even playing "tag" outside with the kids. In addition to finding activities that are both active and enjoyable, there's a considerable correlation between workouts yielding greater success in groups rather than going solo.[268] Examples of healthy activities we can engage in with groups include bicycling, running, lifting weights, or taking a dance class.

There are many reasons for this added benefit seen in group activity. For one thing, positive peer pressure gives us a nudge to prioritize our health in ways we may not be able to when we're acting alone. Likewise, those who struggle through physical metamorphosis together experience a bond forged through "consistency, duration, motivation, conversation and inspiration."[269] In other words, the enactment of community becomes the support we need to carry out actions that would otherwise be difficult. In 1999, the *Journal of Consulting and Clinical Psychology* reported on a study of the benefits of group exercise. It noted a significant distinction in success between participants who joined workout programs alone or in groups. For those who acted alone, "76% completed treatment and 24% maintained their weight loss"[270] for nearly a year, while of those who worked out in groups and received peer support, "95% completed their treatment and 66% maintained their weight loss in full."[271]

It stands to reason that our efforts will be more successful when tackled in a group than alone, and for this reason we won't elaborate. As we've already touched upon, we are made in the image of God and are wired for community, so it's no great leap to realize that we can tackle hard jobs more easily with the resolve of many rather than a few or only one. Here's an interesting thought: If you can't remember how to play, that may indicate that your lifestyle has fallen out of balance. You can rectify this by taking baby steps. Start by trying to recall what you enjoyed doing when you were young. Chances are, even though your body may have aged, you can still engage in a modified version of the same activity—and it will probably still bring you joy.

Another thought-provoking observation is that when we work out in an indoor facility, more internal motivation is required. Why? Because during outdoor activity, the sun actually provides nourishment to our bodies while being outside in the fresh air lowers stress and blood pressure…all while helping us have a more effective workout with extra "feel good" hormones being produced (more on this later). So, while any workout is beneficial, those involving enjoyable outdoor activities and in a group will likely bring you the highest success rate possible. A bonus: Whereas gym membership dues can cost as much as $50–$60 per month or more, outdoor activities are often easily accessible free or for a minimal charge.

One way that I (Joe) look at working out—in particular, regarding how it affects my levels of energy—is to compare it to putting money into a savings account. If I make a deposit (exercise) each day, on the following day, I have dividends to spend. These dividends come in the form of clearer thinking, increased energy, more flexible joints, muscles that are oxygenated, and a better night's sleep (which contributes to all the aforementioned benefits). If I skip a day and make no deposit, there's nothing in the bank the next day. For me, the difference in quality occurs that fast: I am at least 30 percent more sluggish and have more brain fog the day I do not work out *and* the following day. What I'm getting at is that there are many times when we don't feel like working out, but we must keep making those deposits. We cannot "create" a surplus of energy by merely resting on the couch.

When Exercise Seems Impossible

We are aware that some of you have likely picked up this book because you're facing advanced phases of disease/illness that may render the concept of conventional exercise impractical or impossible. For those, I (Joe) would love for you to consider the following.

Can you get to a window? Even if you can sit in a chair near that window, let the sun's rays warm your skin. I encourage you to turn off all media (except maybe some soft music) and look outdoors, taking in the scene that's right outside. Find something beautiful to appreciate in the landscape: perhaps it's a tree, a plant, or the clouds. In a rural area, the foliage and wildlife might provide a breathtaking backdrop. Or, maybe you're in an urban setting, where the hustle and bustle of humanity, with its innovative transportation, the illumination of technology, the sense of progress, and the prospects of on-the-go discovery await outside. Regardless of the view from your window, you can find *something* to appreciate.

After taking some moments to enjoy the scenery God has provided, close your eyes and slowly breathe all of the air out of your lungs. Expel as much breath as you can, emptying as much of the diaphragm as you are able. Then, gently and evenly, breathe in through the nostrils, filling the diaphragm and lungs to maximum capacity. Hold this air in place for two full seconds. Then, smoothly exhale all the air. Again, push as much oxygen from the body as possible, and repeat the breathing exercise three times. Then, spend the remainder of the session sitting still, enjoying the landscape, dwelling on positive thoughts, even praying. By allowing your body time to calmly take in the beauty that surrounds you while ruminating on positivity, the hypothalamus gland is able to dispatch healing resources throughout the body, as we discussed in a previous chapter. Despite your inability to work out, this one habit will increase your health by stimulating the vagus nerve, initiating a relaxation response from the brain to the major sensory organs. This will lower your blood pressure and heart rate, and will help decrease anxiety and aid digestion! (The vagus nerve, "also called X cranial nerve or 10th cranial nerve, [is the] longest and most complex of the cranial nerves."[272])

Try to spend at least fifteen minutes doing this each day (or longer, if you feel inclined!), breaking up time into durations of your own choosing. Begin each sitting with the breathing exercise, followed by the quiet time of peaceful reflection for the balance of the period. (Don't do the breathing exercise for the entire block of time, as this could cause hyperventilation.) It doesn't matter if you do this once for fifteen minutes, if you opt for three five-minute sessions, or chose to do five three-minute sittings daily. We've talked previously about the healing power of thoughts along with the benefits of relaxation, prayer, and meditation. Even this simple routine, done while contemplating good thoughts, will alleviate anxiety, nervousness, and fear. An additional advantage to forming this habit comes from the fact that oxygen is a vital nutrient. (The significance of oxygen, in this light, will be discussed in a future chapter.) Even if developing this one habit is the only change you are able to make to improve your well-being, it is valuable.

If you're unable to exercise, it is our prayer that you won't let that discourage you from seizing all of the quality of life available. You're not defenseless; you have the power to make good decisions for the betterment of your health.

Cellular Health

Mitochondrial Biogenesis

When I (Daniel) was beginning my journey toward better health, I began to recall the days spent with my dad in the woods. I had always known that he had given me the gift of his *time* in those days, but it wasn't until later that I was able to connect the benefits he bestowed upon me by teaching me his lifestyle. As my search progressed, I innately *knew* that spending time in spring waters would improve my health. Strangely, at the time, I didn't understand the science of the process; I just somehow had the instinct that this would be good for my health. It wasn't until later that I learned about mitochondrial biogenesis (discussed earlier). I wasn't surprised to find a biological benefit to the immersion of one's body in clean, cold creek-water, but I was thrilled to finally pinpoint what it was. I was awestruck at the grace of God: He gave me intuitive knowledge that benefited me before I ever even learned the scientific data. This is just another proof that God meets us where we are because He cares about us. As mentioned earlier, mitochondrial biogenesis is regeneration at the cellular level that is triggered by submersion in cold water. The best place to do this is in a creek, stream, or a lake, although the moving current will provide cleaner (and likely colder) water. If you live in the city and cannot get to a natural source of water, a cold shower for one or two minutes per day will accomplish the same thing,[273] but will also expose your body to chemicals in city water. Thus, we restate that it's better to find a natural body of water. There is also the option of filtering your shower water.

How does this connect with exercise?

Many people have access to an outdoor location where they can wade or swim. Others (I know several people) run a trail at a nearby park, then sit in the creek water nearby to give their muscles a natural "ice bath." To someone who's never done this, it may sound torturous, but we assure you that you *will acclimate* to such activity, and the health benefits are tremendous.

On the other hand, a twenty-five minute session of sauna heat activates something called "heat shock," which triggers mitochondrial biogenesis.[274] While it is harder to replicate such conditions in the great outdoors, some places are unusually muggy and hot. In these areas, people often opt for indoor activities with air-conditioning. To a certain degree, this is wise. You don't want to over-exert yourself in such a setting for fear of heat shock becoming heat stroke. Recall that with mitochondrial biogenesis, the key is exposing the body to something that is healthy in moderation without taking the activity so far that it becomes dangerous. However, considering what takes place in a sauna, no one is suggesting you conduct vigorous workouts within such a climate. Instead, after a nice, cardio-engaging workout, you could find a place to sit and read a book or relax outdoors, even on a hot, muggy day.

Telomeres

You may recall our mentioning telomeres earlier in the book. These are caps that cover the end of DNA in cells, and as cells replicate, telomeres shorten.[275] This is the essence of the aging process: the shorter the telomere, the closer to expiration. Healthy telomeres shorten in slower increments, and in some cases, they have been known to lengthen. Because these protective agents respond to the conditions they're exposed to, their health—and ultimately that of the entire body—hinges greatly upon the choices we make and how we care for our health.

The Centers for Disease Control and Prevention (CDC) conducted a survey of more than six thousand patients across recent years. The results were published by *Preventive Medicine* in an article that stated individuals who exercised regularly (these subjects ran for at least a half hour a day for five days each week) were found to have telomeres longer by as many as 140 base pairs—"a difference of about nine years of cellular aging."[276]

Beyond this, telomere length is associated with stress level and inflammation, both of which are alleviated by exercise, thus feeding telomere health in other ways when we engage in regular, vigorous exercise.

Improved Immune System

For many, the link between exercise and immunity may seem like a leap, but it makes sense on several levels.

Micro/Macro Ecosystems

Satchin Panda (the aforementioned executive founding member of the Center for Circadian Biology at the University of California in San

Diego and professor at Salk University) explains that the "germ theory of disease" developed around the early 1900s, when life expectancy was about forty-five to fifty years.[277] At this time, germs were identified as a type of "intruder" that was known to live outside the body. When that "intruder" entered the body, it was believed, a person would become sick. In response to this discovery, the aim became to keep germs out. This was a great early-medicine step in fighting disease that resulted in excellent precautionary measures such as sanitation, vaccination, and antibiotics.[278]

While these are wonderful developments that have contributed to saving lives and increasing life spans to eighty to eighty-five years, they have also contributed to an overcorrection: We're now seeing widespread germophobia, which at times sabotages our health. Eliminating all germs and exposure to them unfortunately isolates our immune system, leaves it quarantined and thus ill-prepared. Our bodies need exposure to germs in order to be able to fight them.

Director and founder of the M Clinic, Dr. Zach Bush, explains that in order to achieve good health, we need to expose our bodies to as many micro ecosystems and macro ecosystems as we possibly can. What do these terms mean? They are used broadly and loosely, and apply to many different fields. For our purposes, the micro ecosystem refers to smaller settings of exposure, such as public and private indoor settings, and macro ecosystem refers to outdoor settings of all kinds. When we live in houses with the windows closed and climate control turned on, and we lack exposure to outdoor air, sunlight, and even the germs that come along with such exposure, we are inhibiting the body's ability to create antibodies that can fight germs.

Essentially, our bodies learn to fend off germs by encountering and defeating them in small doses. Thus, living continually indoors—especially when the indoor settings are limited to just a few locations—diminishes the immune system's strength phenomenally. One of the best things we can do to strengthen our immune system is expose our bodies to the misty air near a waterfall, the clean, cool oxygen in the woods, or even the dank vapors of a swamp.[279] Most of us move routinely throughout our week with exposure to the micro ecosystem of our homes and offices. In order to be healthier, we need to expand the variety of air that we breathe so that our bodies remember how to fight illness. This helps us create beneficial bacteria as well as antibodies.

Stem Cells

Skeletal muscle makes up a large part of the body, and its health is directly related to the condition of many other functions and organs. This seems obvious, but many are unaware that muscle "acts as an important nutrient store and serves as a source of glucose disposal, maintaining the whole-body homeostasis."[280] Thus, muscle health is nearly equivalent to overall well-being. Likewise, muscle bears a large percentage of the brunt of a good workout. It's no secret that exercise—largely because of the muscle's role—improves metabolic function and rejuvenates the muscular and vascular system. Yet, the most vigorous workouts do small amounts of damage to our muscles. This seems contradictory until we understand that through the process of "skeletal muscle fiber repair," "muscle-specific stem cells"[281] are generated and circulated throughout the body, fortifying reparation of other tissues as well. Aside from the regeneration of muscle cells and improvement to muscular health, these cells are believed to strengthen the tissue for fortification against and reparation of future injuries, and they possibly even contribute to coordination, an ability that can prevent future injuries, such as falling. There is a relationship between stem-cell activity and vascular activity, and an increase in active stem cells means the same in its counterpart, which in turn impacts the endothelial, metabolic, endocrine, and other processes while generally improving circulatory functions as well.

In addition, exercise provides greater blood flow to the muscular system, which then carries "oxygen, nutrients, and various growth factors…[to the rest of the body] while carrying away carbon dioxide and metabolic byproducts."[282] Capillary activity is boosted throughout the muscular system, which then benefits and heals the entire physique.

So, working your muscles literally causes them to create their own regenerative medicine.[283] Stem cells or progenitor cells in bone marrow and the muscular system rejuvenate cells, improve circulation, and increase vascular presence, which enhances the amount of and the means by which nutrients and glucose-balancing agents are disbursed. Dr. Michael Joyner of Mayo Clinic said it well: "When you exercise, you get a …[dose] of your own personal stem cells."[284]

Cognitive Function

Lactate is a naturally occurring molecule the body makes during a vigorous workout. While it's known to be a metabolite agent, it's more recently believed to be an excellent help to cognitive function along with other beneficial physical processes, "acting as a signaling molecule in the brain to link metabolism, substrate availability, blood flow and neuronal activity," while it is necessary to organs such as the heart, kidneys, and liver as well.[285] The largest generator the body has for this molecule is the muscular system.

Since the brain has the highest energy requirements within the human body,[286] the need to nourish it is vital. Lactate supplies fuel to the brain, which, during a workout, opens up to take in larger quantities. (Ever feel mentally *sharper* after an otherwise exhausting workout?) Lactate is a neuroprotective agent, which means that not only will the brain be more alert, but exercising has the potential to help retain cognitive function and even help reverse brain injury in some cases. Further, exercise-induced creation of lactate can increase the presence of neurotrophic factors (proteins that regenerate), which can initiate regeneration of brain cells and increase the storage capacity of the hippocampus, which better accommodates learning and memory and facilitates more successful transfer of information into long-term memory.[287] Additionally, Harvard Medical School neurology instructor Dr. Scott McGinnis confirmed that the prefrontal cortex and medial temporal cortex (which facilitate thinking and memory) have larger capacity in individuals who work out.[288]

Such improvements to overall cognition help ward off Alzheimer's disease, Parkinson's disease, and other degenerative illnesses. Since such conditions are linked to cardiovascular disease, working out has a double benefit: The heart-healthy aspect indirectly feeds cognitive functions in later years, while the direct benefits impact cognitive function as well.

We've mentioned that the brain undergoes a detox "flush" during sleep. The improved circulation that takes place while exercising opens up pathways to further facilitate this process as well, meaning that even as you sleep, your workout is still working for you.

Emotional Well-being

Exercise to Treat Depression

While studies have shown that exercise releases a variety of "feel-good hormones" into the bloodstream, thereby improving overall mood (more on this in a bit), it is also true that there is a correlation between people who have been diagnosed with "mood disorders...[and] cardiovascular disease...premature death...increased rates of obesity...and diabetes mellitus compared to the general population."[289] This means that those who undergo treatment for issues such as major depressive disorder or bipolar disorder are more likely to see diminished health. With this understood, overcoming emotional or psychological problems could alleviate odds of developing other health problems throughout the course of one's life. Recent studies regarding exercise have revealed that "exercise impacts both the physical and health parameters of mood disorders as well as mental health outcomes…[and] positively impacts conditions frequently comorbid with mood disorders (i.e. anxiety, pain, and insomnia.)"[290] Activity stimulates receptors in the brain that become degenerate when we aren't active, so, in this way, we have larger cognitive capacity when we exercise regularly.[291] Such revelations suggest that exercise could be a form of treatment for some patients with these mood disorders, showing that it feeds into our overall health in an abundance of ways that experts are only now learning about.[292] It is one more way that we see the decision for good health feeding itself in perpetuating motion.

Feel-Good Hormones

Just the same way that depressive or anxiety disorders are more commonly attributed to a chemical imbalance than they are to life's stressful situations (hence the use of antidepressant pills in so many cases), changing the brain chemistry for the better can offer an effective counter-attack to depression and anxiety.

When we exert energy and our muscles work hard, circulation opens throughout the body, including within the regions serving the brain. The brain in turn releases endorphins—a neurotransmitter that diminishes signals of pain, stress, depression, and anxiety. Additionally, dopamine, serotonin, and norepinephrine are secreted, each of which plays a vital role in streamlining moods and helping emotions get unstuck.[293] In fact, a recent study conducted by researchers at Harvard T. H. Chan School of Public Health revealed that the odds of developing major depression decreased by 26 percent in those who went for one fifteen-minute run per day or a one-hour walk.[294]

Because these "feel-good" chemicals bring about a sense of well-being, we become more motivated over time to continue good habits of working out, which increases self-esteem through improved body image and feelings of empowerment. Additionally, as general health improves, subsequent workout sessions become easier because the body is in better shape. This then contributes to a more positive outlook along with diminished stress and depression. These chemicals, combined with the flushing detox that takes place as a result of heightened circulation, help regulate chemicals such as adrenalin, which further adds to a sense of well-being and stress management. Thus, overall improved mental health is enjoyed, and combined with improved cognitive function, the positive results begin to feed into each other in countless ways.

Cardiovascular/Respiratory Health

One of the first things people think of concerning the health benefits of exercise is cardiovascular health. Working out expands the arteries, which reduces blood pressure, and it causes the nervous system to respond to stress on a more relaxed level, which diminishes odds of developing hypertension.

In addition, exercise accomplishes something called ischemic preconditioning.[295] During exercise, the heart has to work hard to circulate the blood throughout the body, thus returning the same blood to itself. As a result, the flow of blood *to* the heart becomes diminished. The heart is conditioned to tolerate surges and depletions in blood supply without panicking and malfunctioning. Since the heart becomes adaptable to this situation, future encounters with plaque in the arteries surrounding the heart have smaller chance of resulting in fatality. According to an article in Harvard Medical School's *Harvard Heart Letter*, "ischemic preconditioning seems to protect the heart if a heart attack does occur later on…[in life], reducing damage by as much as 50%."[296]

Resting heart rate is lower among people who work out regularly, meaning that blood pressure naturally registers at a lower level and allows the heart to regularly work at an easier pace than those who live sedentary lives. Cholesterol levels improve and the heart is able to maintain regular blood flow, which decreases chances of stroke, heart attack, cardiovascular disease, and cardiac arrest.[297]

As we work out, the heart and lungs must meet the demand across the entire body for additional blood flow and oxygen. And, just like any other muscle in the body, the harder it works, the stronger it becomes. This is only one of the ways activity benefits the heart. The lungs, as alluded to a moment ago, share this benefit as well. For the resting person, breathing about fifteen times per minute is common. However, when exercising, breathing can increase to as much as forty to sixty times per minute, processing as much as a hundred liters of air each minute, while expelling carbon dioxide (the byproduct of energy creation and conversion within the body) from the lungs.[298] As we exercise, we work the lungs, which strengthen as they keep up with the flow of oxygen throughout the body, and in turn, "the muscles of the neck and chest, including the diaphragm and muscles between the ribs that work together to power inhaling and exhaling" are often fortified as well, strengthening the lungs' support system.[299]

Sleep

Exercise is linked to quality of sleep in a cyclical fashion. The better we rest, the more energized we feel, giving us greater motivation for a good workout. However, exercise likewise contributes to improved sleep. At first, this can seem tough: the initial aches and pains of a new exercise routine may impede sleep, while a poor night's slumber may tempt us to opt out of any more physical activity. If we are patient and persevere through this initial cycle, our sleep and activity benefits will begin to fall into sync, making both factors more beneficial. Dr. Charlene Gamaldo of the Johns Hopkins Center for Sleep stated: "We have solid evidence that exercise does, in fact, help you fall asleep more quickly and improves sleep quality." However, she concedes, "We may never be able to pinpoint the mechanism that explains how the two are related."[300] It is worth noting that exercise is directly correlated with greater quantities of slow-wave sleep, elevated moods, and diminished levels of anxiety and depression. Perhaps the increased peace we encounter as a result of the chemical reaction to exercise feeds the cycle of improved sleep as well.[301]

Metabolism

You may have heard it said that exercising boosts your metabolism. But many people are uninformed as to what this means, beyond assuming that a healthier metabolism is always a good thing. The body burns calories in three ways: The RMR (resting metabolic rate), the TEF (thermic effect of food), and the PAEE (physical activity energy expenditure).[302] The RMR is the allocation of energy each day that the body needs to keep the organs and systems of the body functioning, and it accounts for about 75 percent of the energy expended on any given day. The TEF makes up less than 10 percent of energy used each day, as is the energy exerted by the digestive system when food is being processed. The PAEE is energy spent when the body is physically active.[303] Of the three types, the PAEE is the method that we have the most direct, *intentional* control over. It's very simple: If we work more, we burn more. A sedentary lifestyle leaves this variable much closer to zero than an active one.

But, that isn't the end of where our choices influence how our calories are burned.

Many recent studies have sought to learn whether the RMR is secondarily impacted by the PAEE. While the jury is still out, many authoritative sources maintain an affirmative correlation between expending through the PAEE to impact the RMR, which alludes to the concept that exercise speeds up the metabolism—even when the body is at rest.

You may wonder how this could be. The body stores glucose throughout the muscular system. When the muscles are worked, the body uses that glucose for energy to get through the activity. The vascular system increases activity throughout the muscular system. This results in the perpetual need for additional energy to be spent, both by restocking glucose in muscles and via the additional vascular support necessary throughout the body. This means that the RMR uses more calories even when the body is not working out, just because it supports a body that *regularly does* work out. Note, however, that the *type* of workout makes a difference in the change in RMR. For example, activities that use less glucose (such as cardio workouts) don't have as much of an effect on RMR as those that strain the muscle more (thus depleting its glucose by a greater amount), such as high-intensity workouts or weight training.[304] However, even workouts that do not speed up RMR are beneficial in many other ways as noted in this chapter.

Hunger

Beyond the possibility of impacting RMR (thus burning more calories at all times), exercise can be its own appetite suppressant. This seems counter-intuitive; it seems reasonable that more activity would create more demand on the body, which would equal the need for additional energy, which would cause the need for more fuel, resulting in a bigger appetite.

So how does this work?

The hypothalamus is the part of the brain that interacts with a set of receptors in the brain known as the POMC (proopiomelanocortin) neurons, which send myriad hormonal signals—including that of appetite suppression—throughout the body.[305] These are triggered when the body temperature elevates. Have you ever had diminished appetite on a hot summer day? The principle is similar, but much more effective when obtained through exercise.

One study confirmed this when researchers observed mice on treadmills for durations of forty minutes at a time. They found that as the animals' body temperatures elevated, their appetites plummeted, and that the mice "had an approximately 50% lower food intake after the treadmill session than their counterparts that had not taken part in the exercise."[306]

Furthermore, studies have shown that two hunger-related hormones, ghrelin and peptide YY, are secreted at different rates when we exercise.[307] Ghrelin is a hormone-causing element, while peptide YY is a suppressant. An article published by the American Physiological Society regarding an experiment in 2008 discussed university students who voluntarily participated in vigorous workouts while they were asked questions to mark their appetites and key-points indicative of ghrelin and peptide YY levels. It was discovered that those who engaged in cardio exercise saw a significant drop in ghrelin levels, while peptide YY increased. Participants who did weight-training workouts saw an increase in ghrelin, but no change in peptide YY. The conclusion of the experiment stated that "strenuous aerobic exercise transiently suppresses appetite."[308]

How Do You Get started?

It is obvious at this point that the benefits of exercise are monumental. However, if you want to maximize your workout, you can multiply the return on your physical investment by doing it outside, in the sun. Many people are unaware of the benefits of sunlight, or the myriad ways it can further give momentum to our efforts of healthy behavior. This will be the topic of an upcoming chapter.

There is good news for those who get hung up on the concept of exercising thirty minutes each day. For many, finding such a regular chunk of time is impossible. However, Michael Joyner of the Mayo Clinic states that three ten-minute sessions are just as effective. This means that during a fifteen-minute break at work, or just by taking the stairs instead of the elevator, we can begin to enjoy the health benefits of working out. He also states that it's "never too late" and that we should find a sustainable, workable plan that is easy for to stick to for optimal results rather than beating ourselves up over not being able to commit to big routines.

It is obvious that finding a way to exercise can only do our health good. Few would argue this point. However, adjusting our point of view toward activity will improve the likelihood that we'll act upon this knowledge. Consider, as mentioned at the beginning of the chapter, the way you played as a child. If we found as much joy in being physically active as we did when we were children, it wouldn't even be necessary to point out the advantages of exercise. We would do it for no other reason than that we *enjoy* it. Consider that all the benefits discussed in this chapter mean we will revel in a longer, healthier life. Further, weight loss, diminished obesity, elevated moods, and even more restful sleep are rewards that will energize us to feel motivated to continue playing. In turn, the increased feeling of well-being fosters general well-being that would make us feel joyful—even *happy*—again.

We would feel young again.

Like we were kids again.

George Bernard Shaw said: "We don't stop playing because we grow old; we grow old because we stop playing."[309] We challenge you to tap into the vast fountain of youth that awaits by beginning to *use your body* again the way your Creator intended. Just as God imparted knowledge to me (Daniel) instinctively via the need for spring water, He loves you and wants you to live a happy and youthful life. I encourage you not to beat yourself up for the years you may have spent not being active, *or* for any of your current limitations. Instead, I implore you to consider what activities you're able to do—then go out and enjoy them!

So how to start? We have to create space for recreation, then look for activities that get us up and out of our chairs, things that we enjoy. If we approach exercise from this angle, it won't be hard to motivate ourselves. We have to remove the task-oriented approach we have toward physical activity and look for ways to take it outdoors, into the sun, and make it fun again. Even better, it needs to be a communal activity that will strengthen relationships and allow us to bond with others again. We live too many hours alone at our computers, with a beautiful world right outside our window. It's time for us to remember what it's like to play, and get outside and do so, regardless of age.

chapter ten

Sunlight, Oxygen, and Pain Management

After spending so much time talking about exercise, it only makes sense to elaborate on how much better it can be when we take it outdoors, where we can breathe in the fresh air and feel the warm sunlight on our skin. Many are unaware that when these rays hit our skin, vitamin D is produced through something called D-creating synthesis.[310] (Vitamin D is made from the cholesterol stores within the skin when it is exposed to sunlight.) The unique thing about D is that while it is a vitamin, it actually operates as a hormone that interacts with receptors throughout the body.[311] This essential is a key player in preventing many illnesses, and deficiencies of it have been linked to all kinds of health problems.

We've already discussed the importance of melatonin, but many are unaware that "the greatest influence on its secretion is [sun] light."[312] This is because the lack of exposure to these beams can interrupt melatonin production and function, impeding these necessities.[313] With the sun being a primary source of D, some experts have even noted a correlation between this vitamin and telomere length, although studies are still underway. Needless to say, vitamin D is essential; we mean this in the very context that it is necessary for the body to function. While there are traces of it in some foods (beef liver, sardines, egg yolks, tuna, salmon, cod liver oil, and swordfish are a few examples), it's nearly impossible to meet the body's need through diet.[314]

In years past, when society's livelihood was primarily agricultural, vitamin D deficiency was nearly unheard of. Unfortunately, in today's sedentary culture, shortages run rampant because many of us simply don't spend enough time outdoors. According to a study released in 2011, more than 40 percent of the subjects tested were vitamin D deficient.[315] Further, even those who *do* spend time outdoors usually block the sun's valuable rays from their bodies with sunscreen, unaware that in most cases, the damage of the deficiency can be more costly to one's health than a sunburn.[316]

Immune System and Healing

Vitamin D is responsible for fortifying the immune system, so a deficiency of it places our health in a vulnerable spot. In fact, correlations have been made between lack of D and respiratory (colds, bronchitis, even pneumonia) infections amongst children.[317] Other studies have successfully confirmed this link in adults as well.

Vitamin D is considered an immunomodulator, an agent that alters the immune system. Immunomodulators can operate with positive or negative results; in this case, the interaction is beneficial. Thus, it is recognized that a shortage of vitamin D causes the immune system to operate without the necessary resources to operate at full capacity. When the immune system is compromised, it sets off a chain reaction of negative effects that can tax the adrenal system and lead to chronic illness, similar to the leaky-gut scenario described earlier. As shown in that discussion, when the immune system malfunctions, it can even, at times, turn inward and attack its host body.

One example of this can be seen through a study that analyzed patients who had diabetes accompanied by a foot infection. Findings show that the immune system has malfunctioned and attacked the extremity of the individual suffering from diabetes. Since such an injury is associated with an altered immune function, researchers sought to learn if there was a correlation between severe cases of diabetes, an accompanying foot injury, and a vitamin D shortage. They discovered that those with the most diminished supplies of D *also* had the highest levels of a component called inflammatory cytokine, a substance secreted by the immune system causing inflammation as a result of injury.[318] The heightened presence of cytokine reveals a cyclical battle fought by the immune system, which turned inward on its host body, causing self-harm. As inflammatory cytokine mounts, it is revelatory of both the body's *attempt to* and simultaneous *inability to* heal itself. Thus, the relationship between diabetes and inflammatory cytokine in the presence of this particular wound shows that the immune system of the D-deficient patient is unable to properly repair itself, and even its best efforts will escalate into more severe injury.

Bone, Joint, and Thyroid Connection

Vitamin D deficiency has also been connected to back and joint pain, as it facilitates healthy bone metabolism and neuromuscular function.[319] One study looked at citizens of Turkish immigration residing in Germany, with particular interest in veiled women as it pertained to a link between D deficiency and secondary hyperathyroidism (sHPT) when present alongside bone or joint pain.[320] This may seem odd until we understand how sHPT comes to be. This condition is often caused when the thyroid has become overstimulated, often a result of the overproduction of a chemical called thyroid-stimulating hormone (TSH). In turn, TSH is usually the result of one of two triggers: kidney failure or vitamin-D deficiency.[321] And here's an interesting point of trivia: During kidney failure, the organ is no longer able to manufacture vitamin D for the body as it often does to compensate when the deficiency is present. When we look at the big picture, we can see the chain reaction taking place.

Returning to our study regarding Turkish immigrants, the body suffering from secondary hyperathyroidism occurring alongside bone pain is consistent with the link between lack of sunlight and the kidney's inability to manufacture D (or its ability to produce only extremely low levels of it). One intriguing result of the research proves our point: This ailment was extremely common among sunlight-deprived individuals, especially among the women who wore veils, those whose skin never sees the light of day.[322]

In a separate study, patients with hypothyroidism (slightly different than the sHPT mentioned previously) were observed over a twelve-week period to see if those given vitamin D supplementation would see a diminished presence of thyroid-stimulating hormone (TSH), which would indicate lower levels of the chemical that instigates many thyroid malfunctions (sHPT is one example). Researchers saw a significant decrease of TSH. As a bonus, since D is a cofactor to the body's ability to retain calcium, participants indicated a boost in those levels as well.[323]

This shows an unexpected connection between thyroid and musculoskeletal well-being—not because each system is dependent on the other, but because both depend on a substantial influx of vitamin D. In fact, according to one study, more than 60 percent of those who suffered from nonspecific skeletal pain (with pain in the legs an especially common complaint) had a vitamin-D shortage. The correlations between these studies offer hope to those who struggle with these issues. For those with thyroid problems or bone/joint pain, this simple solution—rectifying the vitamin-D deficiency—may provide great relief.

Arthritis and bone loss among women has been tied to a vitamin-D shortage as well. One study linked heightened D deficiencies with post-menopausal women (nearly 85 percent of participants were deficient on some level), and this was strongly connected to diminished bone mineral density, indicating that D was associated with damage caused by depleted calcium in these patients as well.[324] Separately, an inadequate level of vitamin D is widespread amongst rheumatoid arthritis (RA) patients,[325] and we see this by studying the regions in the US that have the lowest rates of RA yet the greatest amount of sunshine. These include California, Texas, Hawaii, and Florida, each of which report approximately one in six cases of arthritis among adults[326] and range from 61–71 percent daylight on average,[327] while many other states with fewer sunny days report one in four.[328] This further reinforces the point that lack of sunlight can greatly contribute to physical pain.

Research also indicates that a higher presence of vitamin D is related to lower chances of multiple kinds of cancer. More than sixty studies were analyzed to confirm this point.[329] These were broken down to include thirty that focused on colon cancer, twenty that targeted breast and ovarian cancer, twenty-six centering on prostate cancer, and others that focused more on genetic predisposition.[330] After the data was scrutinized, researchers determined that "strong evidence indicates that intake or synthesis of vitamin D is associated with reduced incidence and death rates of colon, breast, prostate, and ovarian cancers."[331]

Digestive Health

As we've said, vitamin D has vast anti-inflammatory properties and is an immunomoderator. Thus, plentiful stores of it help the immune system thrive and inflammatory levels to be manageable, while a deficiency can allow immune malfunction and heightened inflammation. Since so many illnesses that affect the digestive tract are triggered by inflammation or malfunctioning immune activity, it stands to reason that high concentrations of vitamin D would have a directly beneficial impact on the digestive tract. This concept is fortified by an article published in the *International Journal of Epidemiology* that explore occurrences of colon cancer in relation to geographical regions defined under the parameters of sun exposure.[332] Researchers noted a strong inverse relationship between sunlight quality in a region and the percentage of residents who suffer from colon cancer. For example, the sunny state of New Mexico shows a rate of 6.7 percent, while Arizona shows 10.11 percent for colon cancer. On the other hand, states experiencing diminished sunlight claim higher rates: New York is at 17.3 percent, with New Hampshire at 15.3 percent, and Vermont at 11.3 percent.[333]

Emotional Well-Being

We also find much scientific support for a correlation between a vitamin-D shortage and depression. This is ironic, considering that society's usage of antidepressants is at an all-time high, with twenty-five million adults currently claiming at least two years of use, constituting a 60 percent increase over the number of those who say they've used antidepressants in the past decade.[334] While this is a shocking statistic, more alarming is that many who take these medications find it impossible to stop using them because of "harsh withdrawal symptoms they say they were not warned of."[335] Yet, the correlation between D and depression shows that the sun is the best antidepressant in the world, and best of all, *it's free!*

The beneficial link seems to manifest amongst members of any age, race, or demographic. A study observing depression in obese patients showed that the connection is present and that increasing D diminishes depressive symptoms.[336] Especially among the elderly, experts have observed this correlation.[337] Other studies also show a link between vitamin D and behavior problems in children and adolescents.[338]

One of the most commonly recognized symptoms of the relationship between vitamin D and emotional well-being is seen in seasonal affective disorder (SAD). This depressive disorder comes about, as its name indicates, seasonally, usually striking in the fall and lasting through the winter months. It is in a category all by itself among other psychological or depressive disorders, because it manifests in individuals who suffer no similar symptoms throughout the rest of the year, isolating its appearance to the time when the availability of sunlight is at its lowest. This allows researchers to observe it as pertaining specifically to a deficiency of vitamin D without the complication of crossing disorders or conditions. In other words, when people are otherwise fully functional and happy, but then experience a rather sudden onset of a depressive disorder that can manifest in symptoms such as deep sadness lasting all day, apathy toward subjects typically of interest to the individual, lack of energy, irritability, insomnia, feelings of worthlessness, hopelessness, or thoughts of suicide,[339] we see that shift as *situational*. At that point, we must ask what changed?

If this shift in personality occurred in conjunction with a change in life circumstances, it would be understandable, but we would see a smoother ebb and flow across the year as we do with many other mood disorders, rather than the spike of nearly ten million Americans who experience this onset abruptly in the late fall, the majority of whom obtain relief at the arrival of spring.[340] Additionally, larger numbers of people with SAD live in northern latitudes that receive less sunlight than those who live in the sunny southern hemisphere.[341] Thus, SAD gives us a unique setting by which to observe the impact of a vitamin-D shortage on our moods. However, only in recent years has widespread understanding emerged that SAD is a byproduct of low levels of vitamin D. In 2017, the author of an article in the *Journal of Global Diabetes & Clinical Metabolism* stated: "During winter, when vitamin D levels are low, serotonin levels decline, mood[s] plunge and people often experience cravings for carbohydrates as a means to increase serotonin levels."[342] This is accurate on many levels. It seems that many people gain weight in the winter months. Some blame the holidays, but we have to wonder if the food surrounding us at holidays is a byproduct of the cravings we're experiencing as a result of our bodies' search for serotonin. While engaging this question further could result in a cyclical quandary not unlike the chicken and the egg, it is (literally) food for thought. We digress…

Many professionals are now recommending light treatments rather than antidepressants for SAD. In one type of treatment, a patient sits for a half hour each day by a box light that puts out ten thousand lux (measured unit of light).[343] Because the neuron melanopsin (discussed earlier) sends light signals to the brain (recall that this even takes place for the blind) that stimulate us for activity, the concept is that the light will boost the mood. According to *Harvard Health Magazine*, this is "at least as effective as antidepressant medications for treating seasonal affective disorder," despite the fact it may not be completely effective for every patient.[344] On the other hand, some are treating SAD with vitamin D treatments that boost serotonin and dopamine and restore positive feelings. The good news is that this type of treatment is very inexpensive. San Francisco Foundation for Psychoanalysis chairman Mark Levy, MD, asserts that a half-hour exercising in the sunlight each day could likely be adequate treatment for most cases.[345] (How much time to spend in the sunlight will be discussed in upcoming pages.)

Because vitamin D interacts with the hormonal system, some patients struggle more with SAD, necessitating other measures. However, once vitamin D levels are restored, other hormones will likely fall into line. Added to this is the fact that sunlight helps lower blood pressure (more on this in a bit), reinforcing an overall sense of peace. It's also likely that sunlight fosters healthy cognitive function. In fact, some studies have noted an inverse relationship between some types of skin cancer and Alzheimer's disease.[346] As the odds of the skin ailment increase, dementia becomes less likely. It seems that further research could reveal that the missing link is vitamin D.

Cardiovascular Health

The list of the ways vitamin D affects our bodies just keeps growing; researchers have also tied cardiovascular health to levels of vitamin D: People who get plenty of sun exposure have diminished odds of dying from heart-related issues,[347] likely because of the endothelial benefits provided by vitamin D-3. This element communicates with the cellular aspect of the endothelial system to regulate nitric oxide, which expands blood vessels—thus impacting blood flow—while reducing oxidative stress to the vascular system, both of which lower blood pressure and foster an overall sense of well-being.[348]

The endothelial system makes up the lining throughout the circulatory system, and thus provides a healthy blood supply to and from the heart. Endothelial troubles are related to many illnesses such as hypertension and insulin imbalance issues, and even to conditions as severe as diabetes and atherosclerosis (which allows deposits of fats and plaques to corrode the arterial system).[349] However, studies—some using cutting-edge nanotechnology—show that D-3 can actually reverse arterial damage accrued because of conditions such as atherosclerosis.[350]

Research conducted in the United Kingdom took certain interest in people migrating from southern to northern Europe.[351] Because, statistically, the Mediterranean countries see lower heart-related mortality rate than the northern side of the continent, researchers wondered this was attributable solely to diet, or if other factors were involved. Understanding that migrants bring their cultural inclinations with them (among them, *dietary*), it was believed that, should this increased health be a result of cultural factors, these individuals should show similar statistics when living in the northern hemisphere. Data was collected and studied by comparison on the basis of who did or did not keep a garden in both hemispheres using blood analysis of vitamin-D content.[352] Regions with the least sun—such as Scotland and Northern Ireland—showed the highest coronary mortality rates, while, in general, living in the north put residents at higher risk.[353] Additionally, the return showed a "north-south divide," citing the northern hemisphere as having significantly more harmful rates in cholesterol and that even Crohns' disease was elevated in the least sunny areas.[354]

While many experts are unwilling to pin down D-3 deficiency as the *cause* of heart trouble, many are more than willing to blame it for *increasing* risk factors. On this matter, an Ohio University chemistry and biochemistry professor states: "There are not many…known systems… to restore cardiovascular endothelial cells…and vitamin D-3 can do it… This is a very inexpensive solution to repair the cardiovascular system. We don't have to develop a new drug. We already have it."[355]

How Much Sunlight?

As with anything placed in creation for our health or enjoyment, moderation is a key to accessing its beneficial properties. With this said, overexposure can adversely impact our health. It's not possible to manufacture a standard recommendation, as sun tolerance is determined by each person's distance from the equator, complexion, and melanin level—the body's natural defense to UV rays. Darker-skinned folks tend to have more melanin than fair-skinned people, who are inclined to burn more easily in the sun. Generally, ten to thirty minutes of midday sunlight several times a week will help us maintain healthy vitamin D levels. Keep in mind that (as discussed regarding Blue Zones) people farther from the equator need additional sun exposure, since UV rays in these areas are weaker.[356] Consequences of overexposure to the sun can include, but aren't limited to "sunburn, eye damage, skin aging and other skin changes, heat stroke and skin cancer."[357] If you have questions regarding how much sunlight you need, it may be beneficial to consult a natural healthcare practitioner.

Oxygen

Oxygen is known as the breath of life. Some people fail to recognize that it's the most important nutrient on earth—an oversight due to the fact that it isn't consumed via the digestive tract. However, an oxygen deficiency becomes fatal the fastest. We can go days without water and weeks without food, but cellular death begins after only three minutes without air. Yet, despite its vitality to our very lives, a vast majority of us don't breathe properly. Additionally, a surprising development in conjunction with our sedentary lifestyles is a condition called "email apnea:" a subconscious response to hours spent working at a computer, which causes us to momentarily stop breathing regularly, and possibly becoming light-headed.[358] This may seem ridiculous, but it impacts 80 percent of our population.[359] Shallow breathing can pose a risk to our health as well.

When breath is intermittent, shallow, or takes place mostly through the mouth, it stays mostly within the upper lungs. This area is prone to hyperventilation and can prompt the sympathetic nervous system (more on this in a minute). Deeper, *intentional* breathing brings the lower lungs into the equation, and they're more accommodating toward oxygenating the entire body and calming the mind.[360]

When breath is shallow or intermittent, or if we momentarily stop breathing, the body senses threat and triggers the sympathetic nervous system (SNS), prompting an instinctive reaction, as though there is reason to fear. The chemical fight-or-flight response kicks in, dispatching survival hormones and adrenal resources throughout the body (recall our description of the physiological response to stress in an earlier chapter), accompanied by increase of blood flow and in the heart rate. Feelings of anxiety swell, perpetuating the chemical cycle we're experiencing and interrupting the overall well-being of the body's systems. All of this can be touched off by a momentary pause in regular breathing.

Breathing is our first and most essential connection to life itself. When we don't breathe at full capacity, the body is unable to properly oxygenate all systems, which limits proper function. The immune system, circulatory system, and brain cells become deprived of oxygen while toxins in the body linger, which brings up the point that exhalation is vital to the detox process, because it's how we expel carbon dioxide from the body. Some studies have even shown that "oxygen-starved cells will mutate and become cancerous," suggesting that improper breathing could increase the risk for cancer.[361] Yet, many experts assert that most people only "breathe at 10–20 percent of their full capacity," causing the lower lungs to neglect proper disbursement of oxygen to the body.[362] Since "the brain demands at least 20% of the body's oxygen supply," little is left for the rest of the body's functions.[363]

The key to good breathing is in slow, deep, nasal breathing that reaches past the lungs and fills the diaphragm. When the body takes in oxygen nasally, the air is screened through a series of filters known as cilia. Not only do these tiny cleaners protect our systems from as many as "20 billion particles of foreign matter every day," but they also modify the temperature and humidity levels of incoming air so that its introduction to the lungs is less of a shock than air taken in through the mouth.[364] Slow release of breath through the nose is preferable because oxygen absorption surprisingly takes place during exhalation as well as inhalation. Further, the outflow of carbon dioxide through the nose has a steadier pace, which alleviates feelings of lightheadedness.[365] (Have you ever felt lightheaded after sneezing? This is why.) Since the nostrils are so much smaller than the mouth, breathing in this way forces us to keep a slow and steady pace, which fosters a balanced, regular supply of oxygen to the entire body. We encourage you to break the habit of shallow and intermittent breathing and retrain the body to do deep nasal breathing. Additionally, do everything you can to eliminate anything that might hinder proper breathing, such as stress, poor diet, bad posture, air pollution, lack of exercise, and not having enough exposure to plants (bring them into your home or spend more time outside).

The nasal system communicates with the hypothalamus, which directly connects its signals to the cardiovascular system, circadian cycles (such as eating and sleeping), and storage of memory and emotion (this is why a smell is sometimes the most sudden and effective trigger for a forgotten memory). When nasal breathing is enacted in conjunction with the diaphragm, it stimulates the digestive system, promoting healthier metabolism and immunity. It also signals the vagus nerve, which plays a role in motor skills and coordination and communicates with the central nervous system.[366] When you steps back and look at the grander picture of breathing and how it affects the entire body's responses, you'll begin to see how food smells trigger your appetite, how scents such as lavender can soothe you to sleep, and even how invigorating fragrances can motivate you to engage in activity. We can't overstate proper breathing's value for all biochemical exchanges within the body.

Hypoxia and Hypoxemia

Hypoxia and hypoxemia are products of oxygen deprivation. Hypoxia is the state of deprivation to the point that essential functions are impeded, and hypoxemia refers to a compromised arterial supply.[367] Each of these conditions can range in severity from nearly undetectable to life-threatening. Less severe episodes, sparked by a number of causes, can produce damage that is subtle and ongoing. We've already mentioned posture, which lends to the concept of email apnea, since being hunched over a computer screen compresses the ability to breathe correctly. Other triggers can be less obvious, such as spending large quantities of time at high altitudes, where the air is thinner.

Some studies have explored the impact of hypoxia and hypoxemia on cellular health, which speaks to everything from circulation to cardiovascular elements and the immune system. One study found that tumors create a tightly sealed, hypoxic environment wherein cells are deprived of oxygen and mutations are difficult for the body to repair or correct.[368] While vascular restoration involves other factors, many of which are also addressed in this book, oxygen by itself isn't believe to cause cancerous tumors. This isn't what we're saying. However, we can feasibly argue that deep, diaphragm breathing will arm our bodies with every potential weapon against cancers and other such illnesses.

How Breathing Affects the Immune System

When we confine air intake to the top of our lungs, we allow our immune response to be depleted throughout the entire body. This is because our lungs, which are vulnerable because they directly take in air and whatever that air contains, are one of our weakest points of defense. By not using the deeper capacity for oxygenation, our immune responses can be stunted. For example, a 2016 study using mice showed that cancer-inhibiting T cells (agents dispatched by the thymus gland to aid the immune system) were suppressed within the lungs due to oxygen deprivation, potentially giving cancer cells an advantage.[369] In the study, metastasis (the spread of cancer cells) is cited as the predominant way by which cancer deaths occur. Additionally, the localized immune response to the new arrival of these cells defines whether the body will sustain itself against the influx of the disease.[370] Researchers established that T cells "contain a group of oxygen-sensing proteins which act to limit inflammation within the lungs…[and] also suppresses the anticancer activity of T cells, thereby permitting cancer cells…[to] escape immune attack and establish metastatic colonies."

At this point, you may be thinking, "Wait a minute, I thought oxygen exposure was a good thing. Why would it suppress the immune response to T cells and allow the cancer to spread?"

The results of the study show an "immunologic" element of the lung that causes the immune system to be slightly subdued within this setting. Why? Because the lungs take in air directly from the outside world, thus must tolerate and flush out thousands of harmless particles each day. As a result, the immune system, via something called prolyl hydroxylase domain (PHD), signals T cells to remain relatively docile in their response to foreign articles in the lungs.[371] If this weren't so, the body's immune system would continually trigger adrenal responses to every piece of dust that finds its way into our respiratory system. However, this exchange comes at a great price. The body allows particulates to escape the lungs and enter the body, believing that the local immune response will govern intruders and expel those that don't belong. For this particular study, tumor tissue was removed from the mice and fashioned into a serum of anti-tumor T cells, then re-administered intravenously, blocking the inhibiting T cells. The mice subsequently were more successful in battling the cancerous cells.

This study shows *just how vital* it is to keep oxygen intake at a level that circulates throughout the body and oxygenates all regions. The immune system is at its weakest in the lungs, and if this is the only area receiving the vital nutrients that oxygen provides, we leave our most vulnerable gateway wide open, and the rest of our bodies become sitting ducks—with no line of defense.

On the matter of oxygen's ability to affect the immune system, Dr. Parris Kidd of BrainMD states, "Oxygen plays a pivotal role in the proper functioning of the immune system. We can look at oxygen deficiency as the single greatest cause of all diseases."[372]

Pain Management

Since the previous chapter and this one have been dedicated to the importance of keeping the body moving, many of you have, by now, likely asked: What if this movement brings pain? This becomes, for some, a bondage that impedes our ability to exercise, which in turn encumbers our ability to achieve wellness. Thus, the cycle of aching and illness continues. It is a valid question, and the struggle is real.

I (Daniel) faced challenges for years after my injury in training, and in all honesty, I *still* manage some degree of pain. Ways I handle it range from simple to continual and complicated, depending on my degree of discomfort. For some, living entirely free of physical hurt may be out of the question, while others find a liberating freedom from pain. It truly depends on the source and the duration of pain's presence. Options for dealing with it range from pharmaceutical remedies to natural and therapeutic solutions. At an extreme level, options include surgery and steroid injections. But we suggest you consider these, along with pharmaceuticals, as an absolute last resort.

Danger of Pharmaceuticals

We won't spend much time on the topic of prescription medications and their dangers. The fact that you've selected our book tells us that you've likely *already* decided to pursue natural health rather than mask symptoms with dangerous drugs. However, we're equally aware that you may have chosen this book as a tool for pursuing healing from an ailment that is accompanied by physical pain, and thus the topic warrants addressing here. Each illness brings along a unique form of physical discomfort and thus necessitates its own type of management. We'll briefly cover a few strategies for managing pain, and, as always, we recommend that you follow up with a natural healthcare practitioner who can assess your specific circumstances.

In our opinion, prescription pain medications are usually a bad idea for a variety of reasons. First, rather than address the core health issue, they simply conceal symptoms, preventing us from finding a true diagnosis of the deeper problem. Pain is the body's way of signaling a problem, so silencing that message allows deeper issues to form. Chronic pain (that which lasts more than about three months), however, sometimes accompanies an ailment that cannot be cured, but rather managed, and the discomfort remains. When facing this scenario, you may think that pharmaceuticals are a good way to get relief, but you may not be making this decision with the full array of information.

When we feel pain, it is because receptors are sending signals to the brain. Many opioid meds block these signals, providing temporary relief. However, the body detects the handicap of these receptors, and after a time, its response is to dispatch *additional* receptors, resulting in a lower pain threshold than we had in the first place. This means in the long term, we suffer *more* discomfort.[373] Further, because the body's endorphins are similar to opioids, the body believes it no longer needs to supply its own endorphins, and may slow production. This not only impedes the body's ability to diminish its own hurt, but it can lead to depression by the inability to create its own "feel-good" chemicals.[374]

These meds are often addictive; prescription pain medication addiction has become an epidemic is recent decades. Addition to prescribed pain relievers often can transfer to the use of illegal drugs when prescriptions expire,[375] a devastating turn of events in the life of someone who, initially, is only looking for relief.

The side effects of opioids can be damaging as well, because they are harsh substances the body isn't meant to process. Side effects can be but certainly are not limited to nausea, vomiting, chills, constipation, infection (such as urinary tract infections), sleepiness or insomnia, respiratory malfunction, depression, hallucination, and suicidal thoughts.

Another reason to use opioids as a very last resort is because storing them often leaves them dangerous proximity to our families and others, which can have devastating results. Teenagers looking for a thrill, relatives who might steal and use or sell these medications, and young children getting into them by accident or curiosity are only some reasons that these medications (if they absolutely must be in your home) need to be kept under lock and key. We recently learned of a family whose youngest child died after innocently adhering one of his grandpa's "pain patches" to his skin. His desire to mimic his role model caused an unsuspecting family to suffer a disastrous tragedy.

Acupuncture

Acupuncture is used for more than pain management, as many professionals utilize it to clear methylation pathways, treat illness, combat depression, and boost immunity. This may seem odd, since most people picture acupuncture as multiple needles "stabbing" them at once. Many have no interest in trying it because they're afraid of needles; others are suspect of its Eastern religious roots. Each of us must assess this method with our own discernment, careful evaluation of professionals, and a careful look at the atmosphere of the clinic. With all that said, here's a little information about acupuncture before we move on.

Skin is our largest organ, acting as the protective barrier between the body and the outside world. Each part of the body has neural connections with the skin. Thus, this organ can often be the least intrusive way of communicating with the interior of the body without having to invade via pharmaceuticals or surgery. Acupuncture works by stimulating certain areas of the skin that are dense with nerve endings. Based on where the issue is, nerves are followed to their strongest concentration in the skin, and acupuncture is applied in those areas.

Acupuncture needles are usually very small, the puncture is often barely felt, and the pricks stimulate the areas of the skin that communicate with troubled areas in the body.[376] Since, as stated previously, the body responds to injury by initiating inflammation, these tiny stabs alert the brain to the need for help along the coordinating neural routes, resulting in the body's dispatch of healing resources such as circulation, immune responses, and pain-relieving agents to the area pinpointed.[377] This method allows external impressions to influence the well-being of "tissues, gland[s], organs, and various functions of the body."[378]

The concept can be very simple, although its many applications entail a much deeper study. Each acupuncturist (similar to Western medical doctors) has a different bedside manner. You may be more comfortable with some than with others. Ideally, they'll discuss your health concerns and create a treatment plan with you, outlining the costs and the amount of time and discomfort/relief you may expect during each session. Especially for those entertaining thoughts of an intrusive treatment such as surgery, acupuncture may be a good alternative to explore.

Cannabidiol Oil

CBD (Cannabidiol) oil is a way of managing pain as well as anxiety and other ailments. The endocannabinoid system is the part of the body that facilitates "a variety of functions including sleep, appetite, pain and immune system response."[379] This system produces neurotransmitters that work with the body's receptors to accept cannabinoid properties and help the body positively respond. In particular, it's compatible with the brain's serotonin receptors, which foster elevated moods, positive social behavior, and a general sense of well-being.[380] By interacting with these neurotransmitters, CBD helps reduce inflammation by diminishing pain signals. Likewise, it has been shown to reduce depression and anxiety while improving quality and quantity of sleep. In fact, unlike its counterpart, THC, which is a psychoactive, CBD is believed to be an antipsychotic, relieving patients who suffer from schizophrenia and similar symptoms.[381] Recalling our previous explanation of the cyclical relationship between depression, anxiety, insomnia, and physical pain, it becomes clear that this intervention has benefits that can work in multiple directions at once. The pain-relieving advantages of CBD are so strong that even many cancer patients whose discomfort isn't alleviated by pharmaceuticals find relief from the nausea and vomiting that accompanies chemotherapy, along with their cancer-related pain.[382]

Due to its anti-inflammatory properties, CBD has been linked to lowered blood pressure, and thus to a healthier heart.[383] Diminished hypertension is another way CBD can indirectly reduce stress and anxiety. Because, again, CBD works within the brain for positive neural communication, it has even thought to alleviate neurological disorders. Some with epilepsy have used it and experienced relief from seizures.[384]

Other uses for this amazing compound are still emerging, but include the surprising fact that neuron circuits are positively modified, which help addicts find relief from the compulsion to use drugs![385] Some studies have even alluded to the concept that the presence of CBD reduces the odds of diabetes in some cases,[386] and causes a decline in the count of cancer cells[387] and the elimination of cancerous tumors.[388]

With so many of the benefits of CBD asserted here, we must now state that a small fraction of those who use it experience such side effects as diarrhea, fatigue, and weight fluctuation. While this is relatively uncommon, it bears mentioning. More pressing is the need to ensure that you consult a doctor regarding any medications you may be taking that could interact with it before beginning its use.

Physical Therapy

For those whose chronic pain is caused by an injury, illness, or stroke, physical therapy may be a good alternative to pain medication or surgery. Since we've already covered at length the general benefits of exercise, we'll keep information here related specifically to therapeutic motion. However, by now we've established that movement is what causes the body to secrete the fluids that replenish our muscles and lubricate joints, thus decreasing overall pain and elevating those "feel-good" chemicals within our bodies.[389]

Physical therapy can be a proactive way to combat physical pain in several ways. The first seems obvious: It can bring physical relief. In addition, it allows us to improve our lifestyle and empowers us to take victory over the injury. Further, strengthening the area that's in pain preserves the future health of that region while improving communication between the impacted area and the brain. In this way, coordination is improved to an area we want to treat with special care. Additionally, the risk of falling is often assessed by a physical therapist before beginning exercise, and if it is a concern, the therapist knows how to appropriately address the issue. This not only helps during the time of therapy exercise, but also assists in increased mobile coordination as we age and can act to prevent falls during our later years.

Some may think physical therapy is the same as going to the

gym. This is untrue. Physical therapists are specifically trained to deal with injury, and they understand how to break recovery into baby steps. Whereas general, unsupervised exercise may compound pain or reaggravate an injury, a physical therapist outlines specifically what we should do and how much we should do at once. Further a professional knows when it's time to increase the level of therapy to maximize the benefit of our efforts.

Other forms of therapy involve ultrasound treatments, a method in which a machine powering sound waves is applied to an area of the body to treat injury or reduce inflammation. These often have positive, pain-reducing results and are nonintrusive, as it's carried out via a machine that is merely brushed across the skin by a professional.

Manual massage and adjustments are another type of physical therapy. Massage therapy is different than recreational or relaxational massage in that it is not done for pleasure. It often involves deep-tissue pressure or kneading, which can be painful, but this approach can provide relief to the nerves and injury deep within tissues. This type of therapy sometimes involves manipulation, manually moving and stretching parts of the body to relieve musculoskeletal pain, realign joints, and realign tissues.

Physical bracing or reinforcement are types of therapy that involve bracing or taping parts of the body to stabilize muscles and bones. This is a very common treatment for athletes. Sometimes it's done to immobilize a body part and at other times to train soft tissue to realign to a new position.

Electrical stimulation is a type of physical therapy that comes in the form of small electrical pads that adhere to the skin and dispense minute charges of electricity in concentrated areas. These electrical signals mimic communication sent from the nervous system to an area, drawing a response from the directed muscles or nerves.[390] This can be to contract muscles that have atrophied or are unresponsive, or it can be done to relieve muscle cramps or spasms. In some cases, it acts as a type of internal massage to relieve pain or restore blood flow. By using electricity, therapists can interfere with negative communication in the body and reinsert healthy messaging between the musculoskeletal and nervous systems.

Chiropractic Care

Since, as we've well established, the health of the nervous and musculoskeletal systems affect the whole body, chiropractic care can benefit for our overall well-being. Chiropractic medicine has gotten a controversial reputation that, in most cases, is undeserved. Many chiropractors are capable, careful, and well-versed in the ways of natural healing. However, this type of care is not for everyone. If you're considering this type of treatment, look for a well-respected professional with a good bedside manner who looks thoroughly at each patient's entire health situation before beginning a personalized treatment plan.

Many people carry stress in or around the shoulder blades. This can impact posture and trigger headaches. Chiropractic treatment can help alleviate this, causing us to feel more alert and energetic, along with being able to engage in healthier breathing that comes with good posture. Additionally, when the spine is out of alignment, miscommunications between the nervous and musculoskeletal systems are more likely to occur, causing potential interruptions to functions relating to the immune system, digestive tract, cardiovascular system, signaling to vital organs, and the body's perception of stress and pain, which impacts adrenal resources and hormonal balance. Chiropractic care, many have found, can help with all of these issues.

Additionally, sometimes back pain is subtle enough that we don't consciously perceive it, yet the muscular system becomes tense. This can lend to overall inflammation, and, by this point in the book, you know fully well many ways this can be problematic. Aligning the spine can relieve or even reverse this cycle, which then lowers blood pressure as pain is alleviated. Likewise, the lack of inflammation will help prevent arthritis. The result will likely be better sleep due to diminished blood pressure and inflammation, which furthers the cycle of health.

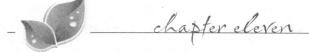

chapter eleven

Embracing the Essentials

The "How-Why" Element

By now, you're aware that the principles given in this book will foster health and vitality in your life, and that these are gifts bestowed upon us by God via His creation. We've thoroughly addressed the "how-tos" of pursuing health through lifestyle choices. Additionally, we've explained the science behind how each of these principles benefits the body. Though we've answered many questions pertaining to "how" these principles are beneficial, for some people, the question "why" we should adopt these habits to develop healthier lifestyles might still be lingering.

Some readers have taken in the practices we've suggested with no need for further convincing; these folks are ready to make lifestyle changes. Others, though, may hesitate, either because of lingering skepticism as to whether these principles will truly render the paybacks we've touted, or because they may still lack motivation to make the changes in their own lives.

A narrow crowd of procrastinators include fortunate individuals who, as of now, have enjoyed good health and suffered no known symptoms of illness. If that is you, you may be thinking, "I'm young and healthy. There's no reason to change what I do just yet." To you, I (Joe) recall your attention to a fact that remained the heartbeat of the book *Timebomb* and was thus stressed throughout its pages: Many natural healthcare practitioners have stated that 80 percent of individuals carry around a ticking time bomb that's waiting to surface and manifest illness. Often, this impending mechanism is correlated with poor gut health, which is usually a byproduct of diet and lifestyle choices. Thus, even if you, as yet, experience no symptoms, I can't emphasize enough that you take preventative action in an effort to keep the level of vitality you currently enjoy. (As a side note, it's likely that you actually *are* experiencing some subtle symptom—acne, fatigue, hair loss, eczema, or unnecessary muscle soreness—that you've simply assumed is "normal." In this case, you may have been conditioned to feel less than optimal and would be surprised at how much better your health improves after making the recommended adjustments.)

For others, there are many potential reasons you may remain hesitant. If you have struggled with long-term chronic illness and feel a lack of empowerment over your condition, motivation may be an issue. This could be especially true if you've already been through the gamut of medications, fad diets, or other trending "remedies" that promised hope but ultimately failed. I (Joe) completely understand this, as anyone who has read my story is aware that it took years of relentlessly seeking medical intervention before I finally found the natural path that changed my life. For those who have walked a similar lane, the motivation to try (and thus place faith or hope in) yet another regimen may still be lacking. Likewise, you may not yet be unconvinced that these principles can work because they're just so simple. It can be hard for those who have endured rounds of pharmaceutical intervention to realize that strategies like going for a walk in the sun, eating carefully, and getting better-quality sleep can provide solutions that decades of medical interventions left unresolved. I understand this, and recall vividly how resistant I initially was to my wife's offers of organic foods and essential oil interventions, and even her queries about possible remedies such as probiotics and supplements.

There was a time when I was certain that if the medical innovations I was using were not effective, then surely nothing the natural path had to offer could work.

With all this said, we believe that one thing is ultimately true: the potential of any solution is completely disarmed if you don't even give it a try. Despite the fact that the principles in this book offer vast health benefits, they are impotent unless you *put them into practice*. Thus, not only is it important that you understand *how* these strategies work, it's equally vital that you answer your own question of *why* you should give them a top priority in your journey to better health.

This takes place when you make a personal connection between what you want—your health goals—with the benefits of any particular practice. In this way, understanding "how" a healthy habit can help you takes on more relevance than being mere scientific facts on a page.

Take exercise, for example. We assert that exercise is an important part of any lifestyle; without exercise, none of us can reach optimum health. Thousands of articles in medical journals explain the scientific facts that support this position. Thus, we suggest that everyone who is physically able *should* work out. Scientifically, this is a proven fact, and few people attempt to debate the virtues of physical activity. However, most people, despite knowing exercise is *critical*, struggle with the personal motivation it takes to get moving. We all seem to know that *everyone else* should be doing it, and it's easy to boldly state this from the comfort of our own couches while procrastinating on picking up the habit ourselves. We can find all kinds of reasons *not* to work out, from not having enough time or energy to not having a gym membership. However, many people engage in healthy activity despite any of these or other excuses. How is it that *some* people find the determination to overcome the obstacles to pursuing a healthy lifestyle, even though it can be hard work, while others seem unable to do so?

Many who exercise regularly state that they love doing it, but others confess that it's hard, even sacrificial, work—but they also understand that it renders long-term payoffs—benefits that are intricate and essential to their personal goals. For some, physical and scientific benefits are the aim, while others make it a social connection by working out with friends (thus nurturing personal growth and emotional well-being while meeting the body's needs). Others may only be able to articulate that they physically "feel better" when they regularly work out; for them, that's motivation enough. The common denominator among such people is that they've grasped the "how-why" connection; they understand *how* the discipline positively impacts them on a personal level, thus they have defined *why* they do what they do, even though it can be hard.

The question, now, then is not for us to continue to explain the science behind the principles we're presenting. We've done that throughout the preceding pages. Now we want to discuss *why* we should all want to stand up and claim these benefits for ourselves, our bodies, our lives, and even our families. Our final commission is to motivate anyone who is still hesitant to make any of the changes we've recommended by fueling their passion and addressing *why* it's so important to prioritize our health.

What Motivates You?

Take a moment to reflect on your life. What motivates you? How do you spend your free time? What are your goals? What do you hope to accomplish? Who relies on you for provision or care? Who are the people you call friends or family? How does your health affect them? What do you hope to leave behind when you are gone?

Questions such as these can take much time to contemplate and fully answer, yet they're some of the most important ones we'll ever consider. Our responses often define who we are.

I (Joe) recognize that some readers are grappling with complicated and advanced health issues, and these kinds of questions may bring about a sense of regret, sadness, or even loss over poor health or potentially unreachable goals. I want to encourage you by saying that as long as you're here on earth, God is not finished with you. You're here for a reason, and you still have work to do, goals to achieve, relationships to mend and tend, and satisfaction and joy to obtain. If you have goals that you set during a previous chapter of your life, but that you're now uncertain you can reach, I encourage you to make revised and obtainable goals, and restart your journey! Today is a new day, and hope is fresh at each new dawn. God's mercies are new every morning (Lamentation 3:22–23), and there is *always* a chance to start a new, more fulfilling journey.

Understanding what motivates us becomes the pathway via which we can connect what we know is healthy for us to do with *why* we become motivated to elevate those healthy choices to personal conviction, making them a top priority. Each of you had a reason you wanted to invest time in absorbing the contents of this book. For many, you're simply looking to avoid or reverse illness and maintain optimum quality of life. However, for those who find the discipline to follow through with the practices we suggest, the underlying motivation runs very deep. I (Joe) find great personal motivation to take better care of my health than ever before because I understand that, as a father and a husband, I've got a responsibility to my family. Obviously, I want my kids to learn to take care of their own health, so I lead by example. My standard of self-care sets a strong pattern for them to follow—simultaneously imprinting these habits in their own lives while they're young enough to adopt them easily. In addition, I want to be healthy, and I want them to be healthy, so we can all share as many quality years together as possible, with an emphasis on trying to minimize the risk of disease.

Grandpa's Legacy

I (Joe) will never forget spending summer afternoons outside with my great-grandpa. Even when he was in his nineties, this man would work outside, in the blistering Arizona heat, preparing firewood for the upcoming winter, making repairs on his property, and tending his garden. He was part of the resilient generation that withstood the hardships of the Dustbowl and the Great Depression during the early parts of the twentieth century. This generation, by and large, practiced the principles outlined in this book out of necessity. Their food was homegrown, nutritious, and organic; circadian patterns were respected and followed; and hours were spent working manually in the sun, assuring that many remained healthy until the latest periods of their lives. I remember my grandpa interacting with us children, engaging in activities with us, hosting holiday meals, and being a viable member of the community. Beyond this, he and his wife had been overcomers throughout their lives, surviving the Depression and becoming entrepreneurs; living out a great example of what it looks like to have faith in God; being caring, compassionate people of integrity; and being hard workers who were able to care for the needy and be founding members of their community. Their vitality strengthened everyone around them. My grandpa was an able-bodied and vivacious individual until, when he was in his mid nineties, his heart failed. His passing was peaceful and his suffering wasn't prolonged. When I was a kid, this is how I thought growing old was supposed to take place: You thrived for several scores of years, then, without extended illness, you simply died of old age.

Normalizing Illness

Unfortunately, many members of today's younger generation face a much different example. Chronic illness is rampant throughout our society, and epidemics such as obesity, diabetes, autoimmune disease, and even cancer have perpetually become more widespread throughout the population and seem to attack younger ages. A pediatric specialist in endocrinology and diabetes says that because of the current practices regarding health, "it's therefore not surprising that the global rise in the prevalence of childhood Type 2 diabetes has coincided with a dramatic increase in childhood obesity."[391] Poor nutrition and sedentary lifestyles, devoid of activity, sunlight, and the other essentials fuel the myriad health issues that seem to escalate daily. Meanwhile, health concerns that are often avoidable with healthy lifestyle choices and habits (such as those pertaining to the digestive tract, blood pressure, cardiovascular health, and insulin balance, just to name a few) become increasingly normalized, attributed to aging or even blamed on hereditary status. As a result, our young generation is populated with people who are unaware of how detrimental their lifestyle is to their well-being; they're being mentally conditioned to embrace illness with no understanding that they might have a choice in the matter.

The worst part is that, because our gene expression changes as a result of our choices, our genome is weakening by the generation. We're leaving a genetic and learned legacy of premature illness to our children, who, without knowing how to take better care of their bodies, may accept epidemics with sad resignation. They have been born into a culture that accepts a life that's less abundant than the one God created them for.

Please understand what we are saying, because *unless something changes*, this is the future our young generation is facing *right now*. Our children will become ill and accept it, believing that sickness is normal and they are powerless to prevent it.

Did something in your spirit just shout the word "No!" in response to that last statement? If so, then congratulations! You've established the "how-why" connection within your own life and personal goals on behalf of your children or loved ones. Each of us, by beginning to make changes in our own lives, has the power to take control of our own health. When we do this, we become stronger, which helps us set a great example of living with healthy habits for those who were likely unaware that illness could be reversed or prevented. We also become more helpful to those in need, better role models, and more solid foundations of support for those who feel alone. We increase the odds that we'll have more time on earth to be available to help others. If we want to change the world for those we love, then we must begin by improving ourselves.

We already understand the scientific nature of how these principles will benefit our own bodies, but we must recognize our ability to help others who are yet unaware that their lives could also be improved. This is why it *simply is not an option* to continue on the devastating and destructive road to illness that we, as a society, have been traveling. And the change begins here and now, today. It begins with *you*.

Someone Is Watching You

What does the media teach today's youth? The message bombarding our kids via the Internet, television, and social media is that there are no long-term consequences to our actions, that we should indulge in what feels good now, with no thought of future regret, and that phrases such as "life's too short," and "YOLO" (you only live once) help us both achieve and justify instant gratification. Nearly all principles that teach self-preservation or self-discipline in any way—spiritual, moral, physical, relational, emotional, etc.—are abandoned for momentary and trivial pleasure.

Perhaps young people are learning to be sedentary, spending long, sunny afternoons indoors watching TV rather than enjoying sunshine, creation, and nature. Maybe they are apathetic toward or unaware of toxic ingredients in foods because they haven't been warned. Perhaps they're resigned to accept less than what life has to offer, because empowerment over such matters has yet to be taught them.

It doesn't matter who you are; *someone* is watching what you do and learning from your habits, whether it's your children, your spouse, a neighbor, a relative, or even a peer at work. What are you teaching these individuals? Are you demonstrating that it's normal to come home from work and spend the evening on the couch eating destructive snacks? Is the example you're setting teaching your children to embrace a life that is less than you would dream for them? Perhaps the struggles you've faced in your own health have caused you to abandon the notion that *you* are even capable of inspiring others.

Don't make the mistake of thinking that you must be young and in perfect health to be a strong role model: Many healthcare workers are inspired by the feeblest of their patients because they see in them a determination and will that shows rare inner strength. It doesn't matter what's in your past or how you came to be in your current situation. What *does* matter is how you move forward and whose lives you impact along the way. Whether you realize it or not, you are uniquely positioned to touch someone else's life. This is true *even if* you've previously thought your own story was coming to a close.

We believe that each of us has the power to show others through our actions that a better life is available. And we're certain that, by inspiring others, we can instill within them the knowledge that will help them stand up and obtain their own optimum wellness. We can do this by sharing what we've learned and leading by example. Perhaps you believe your health problem is too advanced to be motivating to anyone else. Consider this: If you can make *any improvement* whatsoever to how someone is dealing with a health issue, then you will have shown that there's room for improvement even when facing a challenging medical issue. Sometimes the smallest progress on the most severe problems can be more inspiring than easily remedied troubles.

Imagine if, because of your own choices, you're able to steer others toward the free and readily available, healthy elements that God placed in His creation, and they, too, see improvements in their own health. How many will find freedom from illness as a result of your influence? It's possible that those you inspire will find themselves liberated in a variety of other ways as a result of their own improved health: a better body image, healthier self-esteem, financial relief from expensive fad diets or pharmaceuticals, and potentially even freedom from emotional troubles and anxiety. The list of ways that your actions can inspire and help others—even during your own journey toward wellness—goes on and on.

Surely you can understand *why* each of us must engage in the healthiest lifestyle possible: if not for ourselves, then for those around us! If we're unwilling to make such changes merely for our own well-being, surely we can see the urgency in empowering our younger generation to take action. These are tomorrow's parents, leaders, teachers, and citizens; so far, we've failed to help them prioritize their health.

These Are ALL Essentials

Throughout this book, we've discussed the virtues of eating clean, nutritious, and organic food; making better lifestyle adjustments; managing stress; following circadian rhythm; practicing intermittent fasting; understanding the impact of our choices on our health and genetic makeup; creating space; paying attention to cellular health; managing pain, meditating and praying; getting the right quality and quantity of sleep; realizing the importance of gut microbiota, micronutrients, macronutrients, and fermented foods; and understanding the benefits of water and hydration; salt, herbs and bitters; exercise; methylation and detoxification; sunlight and fresh air; and more. We've pointed out and scientifically explained the many ways these issues can influence our health—ranging from hormone production and to nutrient absorption to metabolic processes.

Of course, the undertone of this work has been that we must take responsibility for own health. We can do this by refusing to become equated to labels of "illness" or "imbalance," but rather to provide our bodies with every best resource for the most optimum health possible, followed as a daily lifestyle that gives our bodies time to recover from mistakes of the past.

It's important to understand that each of the principles we've presented is essential to good health. We don't get to pick and choose to select only what's convenient. God designed our bodies to interact a certain way within the realm of creation, and within that jurisdiction He provided all of the physical resources we need to live a long and healthy life. These are all elements within the natural provisions God placed here, and He designed our bodies to need each of them. They are all a part of the laws He set in motion for our well-being. Thus, they are equally important to our vitality, and must all be included in our path to wellness.

These elements are all simple and most are easily obtained; there is no reason not to embrace them and make them a part of our daily lives.

What Is Your Body Telling You?

We encourage each reader to contemplate what you've read and reconsider the signals your body has been sending. Perhaps you previously wrote off fatigue, lack of energy, insulin imbalance, metabolic disruption, sleeplessness, anxiety, or depression as normal parts of life that everyone must endure. We hope this book has given you a new perspective so that you'll feel empowered to liberate yourself from precursors to illness, symptoms of illness, or the onset of illness. For those who struggled with sickness before picking up this book, our prayer is that you find total or at least partial reversal and freedom from suffering.

It could be that some of you know you need to embrace these suggestions, yet you remain unsure of how to find time to prioritize them. Our response is this: If you're spread so thin that your lifestyle doesn't allow time for you to put these strategies into practice, then you *certainly* don't have time to become ill! In that case, preventative measures such as we've discussed are even more important. As we said earlier, our children are currently growing up in a society that normalizes and tolerates sickness. This is unacceptable. We as a society *must* restore healthy practices to a place of high priority in our lives.

It's also important that we remember our obligation to take care of our personal health and stop expecting doctors or miracle supplements to save us from illness, merely so that—once we "feel better"—we can continue on the destructive road we've been traveling. How can we expect physicians to fix illnesses and conditions that often stem from such practices as poor nutrition or lack of sleep or activity? While professionals are trained to combat disease by using many of the latest procedures and pharmaceuticals, they're in no way capable of tracking every variable (such as sun exposure, diet, activity level, sleep habits, etc.) in our lives.

It's simply not possible to expect a doctor to reverse damage caused by our habits that contribute to deficiencies or poor health, nor can we "supplement" our way out of the consequences of ongoing lifestyle choices that jeopardize our health. The *only* way to see long-term, improved well-being is to engage in a healthy lifestyle and continue on that path regardless of how hard or inconvenient it may seem at times. We simply cannot alter the fact that God's laws for our bodies are the only road to finding and sustaining optimum health.

Take an honest look at your life. What is your body telling you? What is your lifestyle telling you? Are you living with symptoms of impending illness that you previously thought were normal and must be accepted? Perhaps your lifestyle is showing you that you need to adjust your habits regarding sleep, nutrition, and stress management. If this is the case, then we *beg* you not to put this book down and go back to your usual routines. Consider this moment—today—as the launching pad from where things will begin to change. If you won't (or don't believe you can) implement changes to benefit yourself, then remember those who are counting on you, and do it for them. There is a world of beauty and vitality ahead of you, if you'll only reach out and seize it. A healthier version of you will have more to give to your children, your children's children, your spouse, your neighbors, your coworkers, and even those in need you have yet to meet.

It IS Possible!

Before picking up this book, you may have wondered if it would ever be possible to improve your health. Yes, it is possible! Regardless of how advanced your medical situation may be, how much you have suffered, or how hopeless you perceive the outcome of your story to be, we can't stress enough you can make at least some improvements. Remember, even in the most critical cases of illness, any small reversal can be very inspiring to those around you. The provisions we've discussed that God has placed on earth, free and accessible to all, were put here to assure optimum health for everyone. Remember that it *is possible* to achieve better sleep, live with less pain, enjoy higher energy levels, and even to go about our days with diminished levels of stress. We do this by acknowledging and abiding by the biological laws God put into place.

Also, keep in mind that we can't choose which healthy habits and lifestyle improvements to use and which ones to cast aside. They're all essential. Imagine what abundant life and health we can enjoy if we fully put into practice all of the information and tips we've shared with you.

Leaving a Legacy

At the beginning of this chapter, we discussed the need to make a personal connection between "how" these healthy principles work and "why" it's important to see them as worthwhile investments.

Why, then, should we adopt these practices? As we've pointed out, we live in a world filled with fast, convenient (but toxic) food; that encourages sedentary, indoor lifestyles; that facilitates the overindulgence of every unhealthy habit (such as neglecting sleep); and that emphasizes instant gratification over the importance of time-consuming investments in health. *Why* should we go to the trouble of reprioritizing our lives to bring these essentials to the forefront of our existence?

We must do it for our own health, but there are so many other reasons. It is for our children, and their children.

We must do this for the future of all of humanity, whose very genetics are being written by what we do with the moments of our lives.

Humanity is at a crossroad. What we—*you and I*—do right now will decide the vitality of subsequent generations. Will we take a stand and reverse the epidemics of disease currently being tolerated, labeled to our youth as "normal," "unavoidable," "hereditary," or "the effects of aging?" Will we decide—by changing society's complacency toward illness, common views regarding wellness, the example we set to others, and even impacting our own genetic code—that we will no longer stand by and allow the health of our youth to be pillaged while they're conditioned to accept their circumstances without empowerment?

We *must* stand up—right now, today—and begin to reverse the trend. We can do this by making changes to our lifestyle, our diets, our activity levels, our sleep patterns, and even our stress loads. We can insist on optimizing our own health regardless of how compromised it may presently seem to be. We can make the conscious choice to improve on our wellness, and we can lead by example. We can educate those around us and invite them to join us on this journey. We can remember when we purchase food, health and beauty products, and supplements that we cast a vote using our wallets with each transaction. We can *intentionally* make better decisions, then follow through on that resolution. We can stop expecting the doctors to be the heroes who save us from the consequences of our own continued poor choices. We can turn off technology at appropriate times and seek activity with friends and family instead of looking to a screen for our social interactions.

Everything we need is all around us. When we observe the epidemic of illness that has continued to soar to new heights with each passing year, it is no stretch of the imagination to state that what we've been doing hasn't been working when it comes to our lifestyles, habits, and nutrition. However, the keys to wellness have been strategically placed around each of us within creation, and God has made them accessible to all.

The transformation to a better life begins with baby steps. Choose small changes that you can start making immediately, and follow through. As they become easier, add new layers of change. It can be simple: All you need to do is assess where you are and what you have, and use that information as a starting point to begin the revolution. As this occurs, momentum will build, and it will become easier over time.

In the beginning, God created mankind; He had a design for us to thrive in a garden where He freely provided all our needs—spiritual, physical, and communal. He created us with intention, a purpose, a plan. *You are part of that plan.* You are not here on accident, or as the result of some chance meeting of atoms. A divinely ordained purpose and objective has been appointed for your life; and what you do with it matters. Your health and vitality matter. Your reach into the lives of those around you is irreplaceable. You are part of the big picture.

And what is the big picture? It is to lead our children into a righteous and prosperous future, to connect with others and enrich the lives of those whom God has surrounded us with, to grow in health and live abundantly, and to spread the good news of His love. When we operate at optimum vitality, these easily become the central mission of our lives because they come naturally.

You were placed on earth because God loves you and has a place for you in His plan. You're still here because He is gracious and continually extends new opportunities for us to stand up and claim the abundance of life that He intended for us when He placed us in the Garden of Eden. God has surrounded you with what you need. Embrace it, and thrive.

An Afterthought from the Doctors

The Choice Is Yours

By Dr. Ralph A. Umbriaco, DC, MsTOM, CNHP

The universe, and all that it contains, is governed by a set of guiding principles, fundamental truths. These principles are foundational to the creation of any healthy working system or environment. If violated, there are consequences. If adhered to, there are sure and specific benefits. Your body is an environment. Where you live and how you live is an environment; and healthy environments create healthy outcomes. However, in order for the internal or external environment to become healthy, choices have to be made and principles have to be followed. Success requires some degree of proper education and personal responsibility. My name is Dr. Ralph Umbriaco, and I was asked to share with you three principles and insights that, over the past twenty-five years in private practice as a natural health professional, have proven themselves, over and again, to be both helpful and effective in helping others create and maintain the quality of health they desire.

Personally, I'm energized that the purpose of this book is to assist you in your health journey by providing you with sound natural principles and strategies for creating a new you, a new level of health and wellness. Once you put them into practice, you will grow to appreciate how well these low-cost strategies and self-help tools will begin to work for you—in the comfort of your own home and at a pace that can work for you. To help guide and encourage you further, here are three key principles to focus on as you begin to work out the strategies outlined in this book.

Principle #1: The Lord Creates…The Lord Heals

It is critical to acknowledge that your body has been designed by our loving Creator to be a healthy, self-healing, and self-replicating organism. That means that there is, even now, a natural health practitioner and a natural health pharmacy living inside you that is ready and able to go to work on your behalf. Benjamin Franklin, one of our founding fathers, rightly quips that "God heals and the doctor bills." At the end of the day, all attempts by man to heal still fall under the principles designed by our Creator for that healing to occur. Therefore, the first principle of health is all about acknowledging and agreeing that His way of living will heal and sustain His creation. Acknowledging the Lord as Creator and Healer and falling in line with His principles for natural health and wellness is the first step in moving forward on your adventure toward health, freedom, and wholeness.

Principle # 2: Personal Responsibility

What the Lord has designed inside of us to "work out," we have a responsibility to "work with," in order to receive the blessings and the benefits that responsible living can create. This God-given, self-healing, internally designed wisdom works best and most effectively when we choose to fall into alignment with His plan for personal health and wellness, namely by developing a lifestyle of taking on personal responsibility; making wise choices; choosing and eating healthy and naturally detoxifying, nutritious foods; breathing in clean, nutritious air; drinking lots of healthy, life-giving water; taking in a good amount of healthful sunshine; engaging in some type of regular, enjoyable physical activity; learning about and working our way toward attaining consistent, sound, restful, restorative sleep; scheduling emotional "garage sales" by regularly sweeping our "house" clean of anger, bitterness, and unforgiveness; maintaining a calm, quiet, and thankful spirit; and being willing and brave enough to seek the Lord's help in creating a powerful, purposeful life filled with meaningful interaction, love, and care for others. This type of responsible, consistent living will open the door and enable the doctor within and the natural pharmacy within to go to work and start creating the new and exciting level of health that you want to enjoy and that He wants to bless you with.

Principle # 3: You Are Not A Diagnosis

Rather than fixate on, defend, or fight your disease, condition, or diagnosis, choose instead to walk confidently in your area of personal responsibility. Decide to spend your time, energy, and other resources to create the health that you want, by living in this posture. Over time, you will prove to yourself that disease can no longer have its way with you, and that, by incorporating the principles in this book, natural health and wellness will be yours to enjoy.

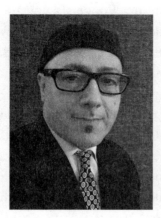

Dr. Ralph Umbriaco is a state-licensed Doctor of Chiropractic and holds a private practice in Newport Beach, CA. He also holds a Master of Science in Traditional Oriental Medicine (MSTOM) and is a Certified Natural Health Professional (CNHP).

As Long as You Have Breath, You Have Hope

By Dr. Matthew Sams, DC, MsTOM, CNHP

At least once a week, we get a call at our office from a patient, spouse, adult child, or friend who describes a healthcare scenario and then asks: "Is there any hope?" This is an interesting question to contemplate. I believe that as long as we have breath in our lungs, there is hope! When man was created, the literal breath of God gave him life.

So how do we embrace this hope?

Find the Best Option for You

One thing you either already know or will soon find out is that there are many routes to wellness. If you go into this with the wrong mindset, it can be very hard. Often, natural healthcare practitioners spend too much time trying to tell you why all of the options you previously sought aren't as good as theirs. This can leave you feeling belittled, tricked, and gullible. This new practitioner will try to convince you that his or her way is the only way that offers any *hope*. Unfortunately, the natural health world has been so attacked by mainstream medicine and Big Pharma that this has become commonplace amongst practitioners as they are forced to defend their proven methods, research, and data against the wallet of the adversary. Don't let their excitement about their type of practice make you lose *hope* or think poorly of yourself from previous visits to other practitioners or doctors. At very least you ruled out something that didn't fix your problem. Now keep searching until you find the answers you're looking for. A patient in our office recently had a major pituitary issue that was discovered by a reflexologist and then confirmed by a medical doctor. Had the patient not been seeking treatment from a natural health practitioner, who knows how long this issue would have gone unchecked? Do your research and find a qualified practitioner who can help you with your issue(s).

Don't Expect a One-Stop Shop

For some reason, patients try to hold natural healthcare practitioners to a different set of standards than the one they hold traditional doctors to. I don't understand this. You would never ask a podiatrist to do an open-heart surgery. Don't expect any practitioner to do the work of another. The same is true with natural supplements and remedies. Make wise and calculated decisions under the direction of a healthcare practitioner. Don't hide what you're taking from any of your practitioners. Certain supplements can have side effects and interactions with others that can be detrimental to your health. One patient in our office recently showed all the symptoms of a blood cancer, but failed to mention that he was on a synthetic hormone, which can cause symptoms that mimic that cancer. It is very important to give your practitioner the whole story.

Live a Lifestyle of Wellness

I tend to make people cry—not because I want to, but because I tell them to do things like cut out sugar from their diet, eat a gluten-free diet, or, remove corn from their diet.

One couple (who happen to be good friends of mine) brought their nine-year-old son to see me about some issues he was having regarding his behavior, his gut, and anxiety. After I told him that he needed to get off of wheat and gluten, he immediately went into hysterics. This can partially be expected from a child, but I have seen my fair share of adults react this poorly, too. Let's just deal with that right now and call it what it is—an idol. The addiction to food, the love of sugar, the belief that we cannot have fun without junk food, and the comfort that food brings has become something that is slowly eroding that John 10:10 (life in all its fullness) type of life that Jesus came for. Scripture is full of references to believers being soldiers. Not living in optimal health and wellness because of poor choices we make in our lifestyle makes it so much easier for Satan to deter us from the ultimate goal of making disciples of *all* nations. We can't do this if we aren't healthy.

Think on These Things

The Apostle Paul, writing to the church of Philippi, said this:

> Finally, brothers, whatever is true, whatever is honorable, whatever is just, whatever is pure, whatever is lovely, whatever is commendable, if there is any excellence, if there is anything worthy of praise, think about these things. (ESV)

The New King James version translates Proverbs 23:7 to this:

> For as he thinks in his heart, so is he.

Countless studies have proven how our mindset can completely change our symptoms. I'm *not saying* you can change your diagnosis just through thought, but God alludes to this in this wisdom chapter. If I could raise my voice at you in this book and scream encouragement, it would be to say this: YOU ARE NOT YOUR DIAGNOSIS! Yes, when you are dealing with your issue(s), it is easy to become known as the person with _____, or it is easy to use your "diagnosis" as your new identity. Second Corinthians 5:17 says this:

> Therefore, if anyone is in Christ, he is a new creation. The old has passed away; behold, the new has come.

I say that as believers in Christ, we need to start acting like this new creation. I say we put on His righteousness and start thinking on the things that are TRUE, HONORABLE, JUST, PURE, LOVELY, COMMENDABLE, EXCELLENT, and WORTHY OF PRAISE. Let me just tell you that your diagnosis is NOT any of those things! Think about that.

Hope Eternal

Ultimately, I have made the assumption that a reader of this book is a believer in Jesus Christ, and this is not a fair assumption. As a child, I put my faith and trust in Jesus Christ and settled my eternity at that time. First Corinthians 15:55–57 says it so well:

> O death, where is your victory? O death, where is your sting? The sting of death is sin, and the power of sin is the law. But thanks be to God, who gives us the victory through our Lord Jesus Christ.

Our world has made death and the end so scary. In fact, the world stands with baited breath waiting for the next pandemic. We needn't worry; in fact, Psalm 139:16 tells us that God already knows the exact number of days we will live. The Apostle Paul had it figured out in Philippians 1:21:

For to me, living means living for Christ, and dying is even better. (NET)

So come on fellow traveler, let's travel this journey of life, for however long God gives it to us, with love, health, wellness, victory, and—most importantly—HOPE!

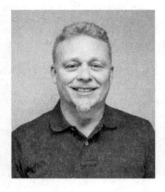

Dr. Matthew Sams is a Doctor of Chiropractic, a fellow of the international academy of clinical acupuncture, and an expert in complementary and alternative medicine and nutrition.

Inviting Jesus Into the Storm

By Dr. Joshua Vance, DC, MTAA

Hey Jesus, How About a Little Help? I'm Not Getting Anywhere!

We often feel alone and confused when it comes to a diagnosis or symptom. Fear can arise and often be overwhelming. Seeking Jesus in any crisis is the answer.

A very strong, well-versed pastor friend said, "If you wanted me to have all the answers, you should have met me in my twenties."

When I was younger, I felt I could do more, believe more, and use my faith more to get what I desired. As I've been through the storms of life, I realized submission is the greatest faith in Jesus I can give Him, and He does a much better job at being God than I can.

John 6:15–21.

The disciples were given a command by Jesus. The command was to travel to the other side of the sea. In obedience, they ventured out and attempted to cross the sea. They were directly in the will of God and being obedient. Again, I repeat, *they were in the will of God.* They had no outward sin that caused the storm, as some might contend. Some were experienced sailors and were confident in their ability to reach the destination as Jesus had instructed.

Jesus was staying behind and interceding on their behalf. He was up on the mountain with His eye upon them. He walked to them upon the sea they were straining against. When has walking on the water ever been normal?

Even in the midst of our trials in life, Jesus never stops leading those who have put their trust in Him (Hebrews 7:25). If you are straining against the trials of life, trust the One who can walk on top of your problems. Get Him involved in every aspect of your life.

When trials come in the form of a diagnosis or symptom, the greatest act of our obedience and faith is to invite Jesus into our boat. Dear believers, does Jesus ever reject those who put their faith in Him? Will He neglect those in need who have "little faith"? NO!

All of us have misunderstood the permitting of God's will. God's will often disrupts our life, even when we are totally doing what He commands. Remember, Jesus has already been up on the hill praying for you in this time. His eye has been on you the whole time. When you find yourself struggling and worn out trying to do what He told you to do, have great faith in Him. Willingly invite Him into your boat. This is the soil for the miracle and manifestation of the GLORY OF GOD!

The health challenge you may be having pales in comparison to His Glory. I know that I often have told God what I wanted to happen through the answering of prayer during the trials of life, but now I don't harden my heart. Instead, I simply ask Him to do His will. This surrender can be scary when you haven't trusted Him before. This is the tilling of the soil of my own heart.

You can be in the middle of God's perfect will and be diagnosed with a terrible ailment or disease. It is not your sin or your parents' sin, but for the glory of God and for you to experience salvation. The affliction can be ended here on planet earth or in the kingdom when you get home. It is the human condition that makes us focus inward on our suffering. I am disappointed when I see people being blamed for not having enough faith or for having some secret sin in their life. Either way, we should not look to our own doing, but to the only One who has the power over sin, sickness, and death. Jesus changes everything.

Even Jesus understood embracing human frailty in a fallen world when He asked for the cup of His suffering to be removed. It isn't wrong to pray and ask our gracious and loving Father to administer healing and relief. Have the courage to pray that God will get the glory through the process, and your part is to draw closer to Him and invite Him into your circumstances, whatever they may be. Not our will, but His will, be done. That's tough, but that's where true faith finds itself amidst loss, sickness, grief, and even death. When the circumstances are life and death, invite the Giver of life and the only One who had the power to raise Himself from the grave.

So, why would God permit these trials? You will not know Him as healer unless you are sick. You will not know Him as provider unless you are in need. You will not know Him as Savior unless you experience His salvation. This is sanctification, drawing closer to being refined in the fire for the Glory of Jesus (1 Peter 1:6–7).

During the refining period with precious metals, the fire is held to the metal, making the impurity bubbles (dross) rise to the top. The heating is continued until only pure metal remains. How will the purifier know that the goal has been accomplished? When he can see his image in the precious metal. If God permits, then God will perfect. Draw close to Him in your time of need and pray that His Glory will be reflected in you. If you trust Him, He promises He will direct your path (Proverbs 3:5–6). He loves you and always tends to you. He intercedes for you even when He seems far up on the mountain. Invite Him into your circumstances and allocate the room for His Glory in your boat.

John 6:21:

Then they willingly received Him into the boat and immediately the boat was at the land where they were going.

What you are seeking will be found in Jesus and much faster with Him in your boat. He is a much better Savior and Physician than any here on earth. Be encouraged.

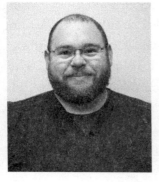

Dr. Joshua W. Vance (DC, MTAA) is a chiropractic specialist in Republic, Missouri. He graduated with honors from Cleveland Chiropractic College, Kansas City in 1999. Having more than nineteen years of diverse experiences, especially in chiropractic, Dr. Vance affiliates with no hospital, and cooperates with other doctors and specialists in the medical group, Vance Chiropractic, Inc.

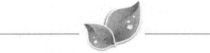

Eden's Essentials

Eden's Essentials began with a vision. That vision was to restore the covenant of good stewardship between our land and people. The place God created for man to live was in a garden. This is not coincidence. It was where we were able to live closest to God free from infirmity and suffering. Eden's Essentials, the name itself, implies that there are things God has created that we cannot live without. In fact, our blessings are tied to them: freedom from illness, a properly functioning body, and good land that nourishes us and keeps us energized to perform our duties and live happily. Then there is the feature that almost everyone overlooks: a complete bond with our Creator involving all three human aspects: mind, spirit, and body.

Our bodies are gifts from God. This beautifully and wonderfully made vessel we inhabit is the vehicle by which we perform all things. It allows us to work, to be good parents and siblings, to honor our fathers and mothers by helping take care of them, and to protect our families. How we honor this gift directly impacts the value of our lives.

In launching our supplement line, the standards we set were first and foremost about nutrition. We decided that whatever we sell needs to be as close to God's original design as possible; in other words, it has to be real food. Not only does it need to be actual food, it needs to have been grown in a way that nourishes the soil and the plant so that they have all the nutrients they require.

A second parameter for our line of supplements, we decided, would focus on cleanliness. The strength of a food or supplement is directly proportional to the health of the soil its grown it. Bacteria, mycelia, organic acids, and worms, among other things, are essential to creating a vibrant, living community. When we spray poisons on our plants and fertilize the soil, it breaks down the natural ecology required to grow healthy food. Furthermore, it blights the land and destroys the ecosystem needed to sustain a healthy environment. There are more organisms in a tablespoon of healthy soil than there are humans on this planet. Those organisms are our partners in making us and the world vibrant and vital. Without them, there is only disease and dysfunction.

Another part of the cleanliness equation is what is used in the products such as excipients (agents that bind, stabilize, or otherwise ensure constitution/preservation of the product) and fillers. Almost all of our encapsulated products are made with 100 percent solvent-free vegetable capsules and vegetable-source soft gels. These capsules are superior to their solvent-based or gelatin counterparts and ensure a healthier, safer product for our customers. In contrast to many popular brands, our 100 percent solvent-free vegetable capsules dissolve rapidly (regardless of temperature) and provide excellent absorption of nutrients.

Our manufacturing partner conducts the most stringent scientific laboratory testing of raw materials and finished products as well as proprietary bioenergetic testing of all ingredients. It has pioneered the use of bioenergetic testing to ensure the customer is consistently getting the best quality worldwide. In addition, it uses the most advanced lab equipment and test methods, including HPLC (high-performance liquid chromatography) to assure the potency and reliability of every ingredient. Our partner's incoming raw materials are tested with pioneering photoluminescent technology to verify that our raw materials fall in our selected "circle of confidence" and are free of contaminants.

An important thing to note is that supplements are tools. They are not meant to replace a good diet, active life, healthy sleep habits, or true friendship. Supplements are tools that we have been given to help us recover the things we are missing in our lives as well as to help us deal with certain situations and conditions. Our future endeavors are certainly pointed to restoring health to the land and our people; in the meantime, we are committed to providing the best tools available. We will remain diligent in our efforts to shine the light of truth on health and wellness, and are honored to serve you in this regard.

In the upcoming pages, we present the Eden's Essentials Supplement Line.

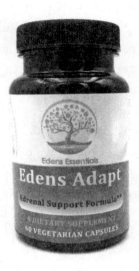

Edens Adapt

- Designed to assist the adrenal glands, which have wide-ranging influence on overall health.
- Formulated to support the body's daily reactions to stress and anxiety.
- Features a broad spectrum of constituents to nourish the body and provide energy.
- Includes a verified PhytoChemical profile (PCPV).
- Tested for identity, purity, strength (where applicable), composition, and quality.

Edens Adapt is a premier quality, nutraceutical formula designed to support healthy adrenal glands. It is a synergistic blend of super phytonutrients and adaptogenic herbs to support and strengthen the adrenal glands like no other formula. It incorporates the latest Chinese research and the most recent clinical findings, producing the super-potent cordyceps formula, Edens Adapt.

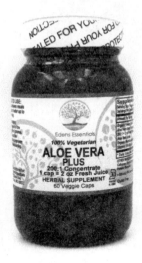

Aloe Vera Plus

- Provides soothing relief for gastrointestinal distress.
- Promotes healthy bowel function and elimination.
- Supports digestion and detoxification.

For upset stomach or colon issues, engage the powerful healing properties of our Aloe Vera Plus. This organic and wild-crafted botanical supplement is a strong aid to your stomach as well as your digestive and elimination tracts. The gentle formula supports the mucous membrane linings and the colon to help ease the bowels to promote a healthy and clean body. Because it enhances the health of mucous membrane linings, Aloe Vera Plus also benefits sinus health and is a great product to provide support across a multitude of systems in the body.

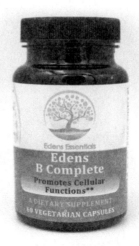

Edens B Complete

- B vitamins play a key role in many of the body's vital functions, such as nerves, brain, moods, and energy production.
- B vitamins are essential for healthy skin and metabolism.
- B vitamins support clarity and memory.
- B vitamins promote cognitive function, heart health, and mood balance.

B vitamins play important roles in nearly all of the body's functional systems. Some of the wide-reaching supportive roles of B vitamins include improving the health of the nervous system, providing support for liver, skin, and hair, and as maintaining muscle tone in the gastrointestinal tract. A sufficient level of B vitamin is essential for adequate energy metabolism, mood balance, hormone synthesis, hemoglobin formation, and nerve-cell impulse transmissions. Because B vitamins work together as a team, a good recommendation is to regularly take a supplement that contains the whole vitamin B complex family.

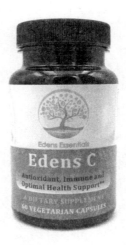

Edens C

- A whole-food vitamin C formula.
- A powerful antioxidant required in a vast array of the body's day-to-day functions, such as metabolism and the absorption of iron.
- A support to the immune system.
- Includes acerola, bilberry fruit, and more.
- Without added ascorbic acid.
- PhytoChemical profile Verified.

Edens C is a water-soluble vitamin that must be obtained through the diet. In human biochemistry, it acts as a free-radical scavenger and antioxidant while providing other important health benefits. Unlike most vitamin C products, Edens C is a potent, 100 percent natural, botanical vitamin C formula without synthetic ascorbic acid or calcium ascorbate. It features our premium whole-food blends of C Food Blend and C Food Support for optimal, full-spectrum, nutritional support. The total vitamin C content in this formula is from natural sources, including organic acerola, organic bilberry fruit, and more. This product delivers premier antioxidant power with natural free-radical quenching activity for optimal immune support.

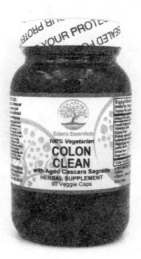

Colon Cleanse

- Assists with gastrointestinal distress.
- Detoxifies the colon.
- Improves overall bowel function.

Edens Essentials Colon Clean is an organic and wild-crafted botanical supplement meant to support the colon and the natural elimination process. This comprehensive formula is designed to cleanse the colon of unwanted matter and provide assistance in the healing process. Many of today's lifestyles make it difficult to maintain a healthy colon. Processed food, environmental toxins, and being sedentary put a lot of stress on the body, and our Colon Cleanse is a good way to give it the support it needs.

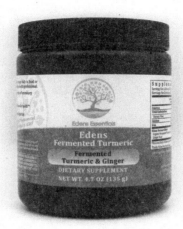

Fermented Turmeric & Ginger

- Fermented to unlock the full potential of this powerful herb.
- Supports a healthy inflammatory response as well as liver and cardiovascular function.
- Assists the body's maintenance of proper blood sugar levels.
- Maintains healthy digestion.

Edens Fermented Turmeric is a revolutionary, highly absorbable probiotic-fermented organic turmeric rhizome and organic fermented ginger powder in their full-spectrum state, cultivated with our partner's signature probiotic-fermented delivery system. This provides maximum bioavailability, digestion, and absorption. For centuries, turmeric has been the quintessential herb choice for promoting liver health, maintaining healthy digestion, supporting a healthy inflammatory response, and enhancing cardiovascular health.

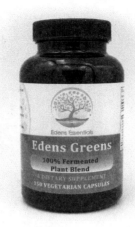

Edens Greens

- Fermented whole foods to assist with digestion and elimination.
- A full spectrum of naturally occurring vitamins and minerals.
- Assistance to the body's organs, including the liver and colon, in detoxification.
- Pre-digested nutrients that are more bioavailable, making them better assimilated by the body.
- Prebiotic, probiotic, and postbiotic activity.

Eden's Greens is a complete, whole-food formula that contains fermented organic barley grass, fermented organic oat grass, fermented organic kale, and fermented organic chlorella, among other superfoods. In addition to grasses, dark leafy vegetables, herbs, and more, it offers a powerhouse of prebiotic, probiotic, and postbiotic activity.

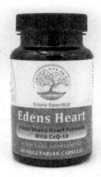

Edens Heart

- Multi-nutrient formula provides cardiovascular support.
- Supports cellular energy production.
- Naturally fermented CoQ-10; fFat soluble in its most bioavailable form.
- Supports cardiovascular health.
- PhytoChemical profile verified (PCPV).
- Tested for identity, purity, strength, and composition.

Edens Heart is a targeted nutraceutical formula that promotes vital cardiovascular health. This product features premier quality coenzyme Q-10 (50 mg/cap), which is derived from a natural fermentation process (not synthetic CoQ-10). This form of CoQ-10 is fat-soluble and is identical to the CoQ-10 that is naturally produced by cells in the body. Live-source, "trans" isomer CoQ-10 is preferred to synthetic, "cis" isomer CoQ-10 in long term use. CoQ-10 is an essential nutrient that is a vital component of cellular energy production. CoQ-10 is an important part of the mitochondrial electron transport system and supplies cellular energy support to all cells of the body. It especially supports the heart muscle and other bodily tissues that have high energy needs. Edens Heart also features two key nutraceutical blends, CardioPlex and Cardio Essentials, which offer a broad range of biocompatible botanical agents with a complex phytochemical profile for additional nutritional support.

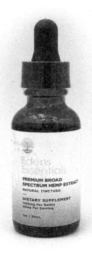
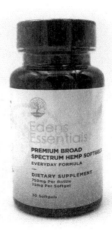

Edens Hemp Extract

- Promotes brain, nerve, and hormonal health.
- Is THC free.
- Can support deep sleep and may provide protection against stress and anxiety.

CBD is a powerful plant extract that has been used for wellness for thousands of years. Our CBD is derived from a specific strain of the hemp plant. It is one of many cannabinoids in hemp that has a variety of effects on our body's endocannabinoid system. We actually have receptors and compounds in our bodies that interact with the compounds that naturally occur in hemp.

Not all hemp is created equal, which means not all CBD is the same. At Edens Essentials, we believe that if you want to create the best products available, excellence must be a priority at every stage. With this as a guidepost, we partner with the right people and companies to achieve a high standard of business. To further our mission of creating the world's best CBD products, we choose our partners very carefully. After extensive due diligence, Edens Essentials decided to partner with the broker of the largest grower, manufacturer, and distributor of hemp-derived phytocannabinoids in the US. This partner makes the raw hemp compounds we use in our products.

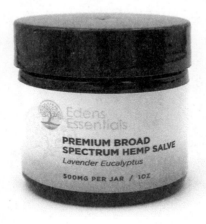

Edens Hemp Salve

Support well-functioning joints with the help of our CBD Salve. A balanced combination of phytocannabinoid-rich hemp oil, beeswax, and aromatic essential oils helps soothe muscles and support skin health.

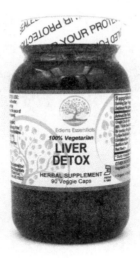

Edens Liver Detox

- Supports proper detoxification of the liver.
- Improves digestion and the regulation of fat.
- Enhances metabolic function and weight control.

Everyone needs a little help now and again, and that is especially true for our friend, the liver. Cleansing your liver is not just for people who like alcohol; everybody's liver gets burdened over time. Liver detox is a moderate-support formula for cleansing and assisting the liver. The liver has a multitude of jobs and is under a lot of stress from different sources, such as environmental stress and toxins, so it is good to give it a hand now and again. This formula aids with detoxification and proper metabolic function and helps reduce oxidative stress. The burden placed upon our organs over time is how we age; healthy choices can help us turn back the clock.

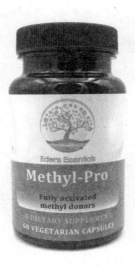

Edens Methyl-Pro

- Supports healthy methylation, neurological, cardiovascular, and emotional health.
- Contains choline, which supports synthesis of a key neurotransmitter, supports cell membrane health as well cholesterol and fat metabolization.
- Contains fully activated methyl donors.
- Contains 5-methyltetrahydrofolate, B12 as methylcobalamin, choline bitartrate, and B6 as pyridoxal-5-phosphate.
- Is quality tested for identity, purity, strength, and composition.

This ideal, daily nutritional formula for the entire family is a once-living phytonutrient formula. This all-in-one supplement provides broad-spectrum, premier nutrition delivering a quantum shift in energy, health, and vitality. We believe that a whole nutrient formula and its entire biocompatible nutritional symphony is priceless in terms of supporting overall health. Thus, attempting to measure a live-source formula on the same RDA scale as synthetics is really meaningless.

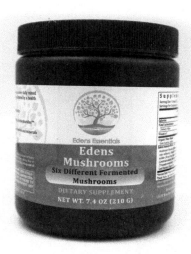

Edens Mushrooms

- Mushrooms offer wide-ranging immune support and are fermented to unlock the full potential of such nutrients as beta glucans.
- The fermentation process means that this product supports digestion and microflora with prebiotic fiber.
- Polysaccharides, powerful immunomodulators, help nourish and strengthen the body's immune system.

Edens Mushrooms feature six types of organically grown, premiere quality, fermented mushrooms in their full-spectrum state. This blend is ideal for maximum bioavailability, digestion, and absorption. Current research shows that the human immune system can be given excellent support by using a mixture of polysaccharides from several proven immunomodulating mushrooms. The pre-digested, fermented, organic mushrooms in this product offer a vast array of naturally occurring vitamins, minerals, and immunomodulating polysaccharides.

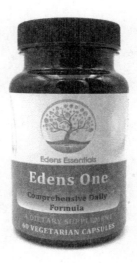

Edens One

- An ideal, all in one multi-nutrient formula for the whole family.
- A once-living phytonutrient formula coming from whole foods.
- Provides daily support for energy, immunity, and digestion.
- Is a phytonutrient formula.
- Is phytoforensic screened for adulterants.
- Is tested for identity, purity, strength, and composition.

This ideal, daily nutritional formula for the entire family is a once-living phytonutrient formula. This all-in-one supplement provides broad-spectrum, premier nutrition delivering a quantum shift in energy, health, and vitality. We believe that a whole-nutrient formula and its entire biocompatible nutritional symphony is priceless in terms of supporting overall health. Thus, attempting to measure a live-source formula on the same RDA scale as synthetics is really meaningless.

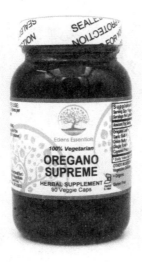

Edens Oregano Supreme

- Provides support for the immune system.
- Is a phenolic compound that has shown antimicrobial, antifungal, and antibacterial properties.

Need some help with immunity or maybe an overgrowth of fungus? Edens Essentials Oregano Supreme is a multi-layered formula containing phenolic compounds that have shown many antimicrobial, antifungal, and antibacterial properties. This combination of immune-assisting botanicals is a good addition to your health protocol. Carvacrol, one of the compounds in oregano that shows a strong antioxidant function, can be a powerful tool in supporting immunity.

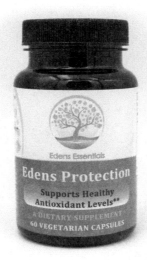

Edens Protection

- Contains astaxanthin, a powerful carotenoid antioxidant, and helps neutralize free radicals.
- Supports cardiovascular, brain, eye, and skin health.
- Is an algae-based astaxanthin.
- Promotes cardiovascular and eye health.
- Quality tested for identity, purity, composition, and strength.

Edens Protection is a unique formula that features a selected range of valued botanicals including natural algae-sourced astaxanthin, a potent, lipid-soluble, carotenoid antioxidant that helps neutralize free radicals. This comprehensive formula also includes Asta-Active Blend, a botanical support blend composed of high value herbal agents that offers a complex phytonutrient profile for added nutritional support.

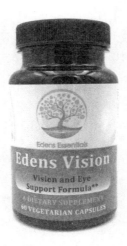

Edens Vision

- Powerful eye and vision-support formula, including the macula.
- Natural sources of zeaxanthin and lutein. Powerful carotenoids stored in the macula may promote the density and integrity of the macular pigment.
- Features researched eye-support nutrients: natural-source lutein (from marigold flowers) at 10 mg/cap and natural-source zeaxanthin (from marigold flowers) at 2 mg/cap.
- Quality tested for identity, purity, composition, and strength where applicable.

Edens Vision: Lutein and zeaxanthin are the two key carotenoid pigments stored in the macula and may promote the integrity and density of the macular pigment through their antioxidant properties. Increased intake of these carotenoids maintain healthy photoreceptor function in the macula as well as supporting the health of the retina. The combination of lutein and zeaxanthin promote total retinal health, photoreceptor health, and overall support for the macula. In addition to the science-backed foundation of zeaxanthin and lutein, this proprietary nutraceutical formula also features 350 mg of the botanical powerhouse, Eye Integrity Support Blend.

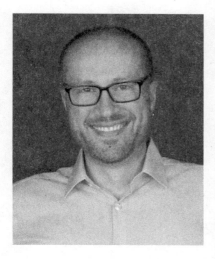

Joe Ardis Horn is a professional fitness and nutrition specialist, COO of SkyWatch TV, dog behavior expert and certified professional trainer/instructor. As the best-selling author of the groundbreaking books, *Dead Pets Don't Lie* and *Timebomb*, his incredible personal story—from the gates of death and back again—prompted the journey behind the development of Edens Essentials.

Daniel Belt is a CHHC (Certified Holistic Health Coach) through the Institute for Integrative Nutrition, accredited by New York State University, and has twenty years of experience in the health and supplements industry. A former soldier, he spent five years in the US Army. Daniel's experiences led him to seek out natural methods that supported his own physical healing, better equipping him to help and serve others with their health.

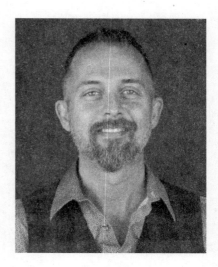

Notes

1. Horn, Joe & Anderson, Allie. *Timebomb: A Genocide of Deadly Processed Foods!* Crane, MO: Defender Publishing, 2018. Pg. 22–23

2. National Institute of Diabetes and Digestive and Kidney Diseases. "Overweight & Obesity Statistics." 2019. Accessed January 10, 2020. https://www.niddk.nih.gov/health-information/health-statistics/ overweight-obesity.

3. Grieve, Carol. "Leaky Gut: Is It Becoming an Epidemic?" *Food Integrity Now*, 27 May 2015, http://foodintegritynow.org/2015/05/27/leaky-gut-is-it-becoming-an-epidemic/. Accessed 3 Jan. 2018.

4. Bob Marley and the Wailers. "Exodus." Recorded 1977. Track 5 on *Exodus*. Island Records: Island Studios, London. LP.

5. Bob Marley and the Wailers. "Get Up Stand Up." Recorded 1973. Track 8 on *Live '73—Paul's Mall, Boston MA.* Klondike Records. LP.

6. Ibid.

7. Tedx Talks. "Intermittent Fasting: Transformational Technique." May 15, 2019. YouTube Video, 12:44. Retrieved March 12, 2020. https://www.youtube.com/watch?v=A6Dkt7zyImk.

8. Griggs, Richard. *Psychology: A Concise Introduction, 5th Ed.* (New York, NY: Worth Publishers, 2017), Pg. 383.

9. Ibid.

10. Ibid., Pg. 384.

11. Ibid.

12. Ibid., Pg. 386.

13. Ibid., Pg. 387.

14. Ibid., Pg. 388.

15. Ibid.

16. Parkash, Vinita. "The Cost of Assuming Your Doctor Knows Best." November 13, 2017. *Cognoscenti Online*. Retrieved April 23, 2020. https://www.wbur.org/cognoscenti/2017/11/13/diagnostic-medical-error-mistake-vinita-parkash.

17. Ibid.

18. Ibid.

19. Ibid.

20. "Commonly Used Antibiotics May Lead to Heart Problems." *University of British Columbia*. September 10, 2019. Retrieved April 23, 2020. https://www.sciencedaily.com/releases/2019/09/190910154710.htm.

21. "Common Antibiotics May Be Linked to Temporary Mental Confusion." *American Academy of Neurology*. February 17, 2016. Retrieved April 23, 2020. https://www.aan.com/PressRoom/Home/PressRelease/1433.

22. "Antibiotic Use Linked to Crohn's Disease." *Health 24*. April 26, 2017. Retrieved April 23, 2020. https://www.health24.com/Medical/Digestive-health/Crohns-disease/Antibiotic-use-linked-to-Crohns-disease-20120721.

23. Rich Roll. "GMOs, Glyphosate & Gut Health." March 11, 2018. YouTube Video, 1:42:13. https://www.youtube.com/watch?v=jWgnkgYtqnw. Accessed January 8, 2020.

24. *Funk & Wagnall's Standard Reference Encyclopedia: Volume 8*. (1959), s.v. "Dust Bowl." (New York: Standard References Works Publishing Company), 2910.

25. Ibid., Pg. 2911.

26. Ibid.

27. Ibid.

28. Ibid.

29. Ibid., Pg. 2912.

30. Aoghs.org. "Big Inch Pipelines of WWII." July 29, 2019. Accessed January 9, 2020. https://aoghs.org/petroleum-in-war/oil-pipelines-2/.

31. Hunt, Janet. "Harmful Effects of Chemical Fertilizers." 2019. *Hunker. com*. Accessed January 9, 2020. https://www.hunker.com/12401292/harmful-effects-of-chemical-fertilizers.

32. Rich Roll. "Food Independence & Planetary Evolution: Zach Bush, MD." January 8, 2019. YouTube Video, 1:54:31. https://www.youtube.com/watch?v=X3aOQ0N74PI. Accessed January 9, 2020.

33. Rich Roll. "GMOs, Glyphosate & Gut Health." Accessed January 8, 2020.

34. Hunt, "Harmful Effects." Accessed January 9, 2020.

35. Roll. "GMOs, Glyphosate & Gut Health." Accessed January 8, 2020.

36. Hunt, "Harmful Effects." Accessed January 9, 2020.

37. Roll, "GMOs, Glyphosate & Gut Health." Accessed January 8, 2020.

38. Ibid.

39. Ibid.

40. Ibid.

41. Horn & Anderson, *Timebomb*. Pg. 40.

42. Kamb, Steve. "Why Sugar Is the Worst Thing Ever for You. Seriously. Ever." *Nerd Fitness*, https://www.nerdfitness.com/blog/everything-you-need-to-know-about-sugar/. Accessed December 19, 2017.

43. Ibid.

44. Horn & Anderson, *Timebomb*. Pg. 98–99.

45. Kessler, David. *The End of Overeating*. (Emmaus, PA: Rodale Publishers, 2009), Pg. 9.

46. Ibid., Pg. 206.

47. Sboros, Marika. "Placebo Power—When Belief Is More Powerful Medicine Than Drugs." *Biznews Online*. March 12, 2014. Retrieved April 23, 2020. https://www.biznews.com/health/2014/03/12/placebo-power-proves-belief-powerful-medicine.

48. Garry, Maryanne. "The Power of Suggestion: What We Expect Influences Our Behavior, for Better or Worse." *Association for Psychological Science*. June 6, 2012. Accessed March 4, 2020. https://www.psychologicalscience.

org/news/releases/the-power-of-suggestion-what-we-expect-influences-our-behavior-for-better-or-worse.html.

49. Ibid.

50. Ibid.

51. Murray, Bridget. "Countering the Power of Suggestion." *Monitor*, June 2002. Vol. 33. No. 6. P. 56. As Retrieved from *American Psychological Association* on March 4, 2020. https://www.apa.org/monitor/jun02/countering.

52. Ibid.

53. Cherry, Kendra. "What Is the Negativity Bias?" *Verywell Mind Online*. April 14, 2020. Retrieved April 23, 2020. https://www.verywellmind.com/negative-bias-4589618.

54. Ibid.

55. Seladi-Schulman, Jill. "What Part of the Brain Controls Emotions?" *Healthline Online*. July 23, 2018. Retrieved April 23, 2020. https://www.healthline.com/health/what-part-of-the-brain-controls-emotions#love.

56. Ibid.

57. Ibid.

58. Mercola, Joseph. "How to Wean Yourself Off Processed Foods in 7 Steps." *Mercola Online*, 1 July 2010, https://articles.mercola.com/sites/articles/archive/2010/07/01/wean-yourself-off-processed-foods-in-7-steps.aspx. Accessed 18 Dec. 2017.

59. Horn & Anderson, *Timebomb*. Pg. 77–78.

60. "Tithes and Offerings: Your Questions, Answered." *Dave Ramsey Online*. 2020. Retrieved March 16, 2020. https://www.daveramsey.com/blog/daves-advice-on-tithing-and-giving.

61. "How to Get Out of Debt with the Debt Snowball Plan." *Dave Ramsey Online*. 2020. Retrieved March 11, 2020. https://www.daveramsey.com/blog/get-out-of-debt-with-the-debt-snowball-plan.

62. Ferreira, Stacey. "The Happiness Value of Work-life Balance." *Inc.com*. February 16, 2018. Accessed January 28, 2020. https://www.inc.com/stacey-ferreira/the-happiness-value-of-work-life-balance.html.

NOTES

63. Ibid.

64. Ibid.

65. Buettner, Dan. "Discover the Happiness Zones Around the World." *Diplomatic Courier* 11, no. 3 (2017): 14–16.

66. Ibid.

67. Ibid.

68. Ibid.

69. Pappas, Gregory. "Remembering Stamatis Moraitis: The Man Who (Almost) Forgot to Die." *PappasPost Online*. February 3, 2018. Accessed January 29, 2020. https://www.pappaspost.com/remembering-stamatis-moraitis-man-who-almost-forgot-die/.

70. Buettner, 14–16.

71. Ibid.

72. Ibid.

73. Ibid.

74. Ibid.

75. Ibid.

76. Gulli, C. "Secrets to Longevity." *Maclean's,* 121(20/21) pg. 60. 2008. Accessed January 29, 2020. Retrieved from http://eres.regent.edu:2048/login?url=http://search.ebscohost.com/login.aspx?.

77. Fischer, Kristen. "Screen Time Hurts More Than Kids' Eyes." *Healthline Online*. October 12, 2015. Retrieved April 23, 2020. https://www.healthline.com/health-news/screen-time-hurts-more-than-kids-eyes-101215#1.

78. Ibid.

79. Ibid.

80. Ibid.

81. Anderson, Allie. *Unscrambling the Millennial Paradox.* (Crane, MO: Defender Publishing, 2018), Pg. 79.

82. "Television and Children." *University of Michigan: Michigan Medicine.* Accessed January 4, 2019. http://www.med.umich.edu/yourchild/topics/tv.

83. Anderson, *Millennial Paradox.* Pg. 84–85.

84. Berk, Laura. *Development Through the Lifespan.* (Hoboken: New Jersey: Pearson Education, 2018), Pg 217.

85. Ibid.

86. Anderson, *Millennial Paradox,* Pg. 89.

87. Dunckley, Victoria. "Gray Matters: Too Much Screen Time Damages the Brain." *Psychology Today.* February 27, 2019. Retrieved April 7, 2020. https://www.psychologytoday.com/us/blog/mental-wealth/201402/gray-matters-too-much-screen-time-damages-the-brain.

88. Graham, Judith and Forstadt, Leslie. "How Television Viewing Affects Children." *Extension: University of Maine.* 2011. https://extension.umaine.edu/publications/4100e/. Last Accessed January 4, 2019.

89. "Social Isolation, Loneliness in Older People Pose Health Risks." *National Institute on Aging Online.* April 23, 2019. Accessed January 28, 2020. https://www.nia.nih.gov/news/social-isolation-loneliness-older-people-pose-health-risks.

90. Ibid.

91. Ibid.

92. Editorial Advisory Board. "Editorial: Meals on Wheels Serves Greater Good." *The Garden City Telegram Online.* October 14, 2019. Accessed January 28, 2020. https://www.gctelegram.com/opinion/20191014/editorial-meals-on-wheels-serves-greater-good.

93. "Social Isolation, Loneliness in Older People Pose Health Risks." *National Institute on Aging Online.* April 23, 2019. Accessed January 28, 2020. https://www.nia.nih.gov/news/social-isolation-loneliness-older-people-pose-health-risks.

94. Novotney, Amy. "Social Isolation: It Could Kill You." *American Psychological Association.* May 2019, Vol. 50, No. 5, pg. 32. Accessed January 28, 2020. https://www.apa.org/monitor/2019/05/ce-corner-isolation.

95. Ibid.

96. Alegria-Torres, Jorge; Baccarelli, Andrea; & Bollati, Valentina. "Epigenetics and Lifestyle." *NCBI US National Library of Medicine: National Institute of Health.* August 26, 2013. Accessed January 29, 2020. https://www.ncbi.nlm.nih.gov/pmc/articles/PMC3752894/.

97. Long, Jeremy; Tymoczko, John; & Stryer, Lubert. *Biochemistry, 5ᵗʰ Ed.* (New York: WH Freeman, 2002). Ch. 17. Retrieved on March 4, 2020. https://www.ncbi.nlm.nih.gov/books/NBK21163/.

98. Serious Science. "The Role of Mitochondria in Aging and Disease." March 6, 2014. YouTube Video: 13:27. Retrieved March 4, 2020. https://www.youtube.com/watch?v=v3ncUYKme4k.

99. Ibid.

100. Dabrowska, Aleksandra; Venero, Jose Luis; Iwasawa; et. al. "PGC-1a Controls Mitochondrial Biogenesis and Dynamics in Lead-induced Neurotoxicity." *US National Library of Medicine.* September, 2015. Accessed March 4, 2020. https://www.ncbi.nlm.nih.gov/pmc/articles/PMC4600622/.

101. Schiffman, Richard. "Why People Who Pray Are Healthier Than Those Who Don't." *Huffpost Online.* January 18, 2012. Accessed January 28, 2020. https://www.huffpost.com/entry/why-people-who-pray-are-heathier_b_1197313.

102. Ibid.

103. Wommack, Keith. "Column: Do You Have a Healthy Attitude?" *Midlothian Mirror.* September 17, 2013. Accessed January 28, 2020. https://www.midlothianmirror.com/article/20130917/Opinion/309179969.

104. Walker, Matthew. *Why We Sleep: Unlocking the Power of Sleep and Dreams.* (New York: Scribner, 2017), Pg.14.

105. Ibid., Pg. 18.

106. Ibid., Pg. 22.

107. Ibid., Pg. 20.

108. Oaklander, Mandy. "This Is Your Brain on 10 Years of Working the Night Shift." *Time Magazine Online.* November 4, 2014. Accessed February 3, 2020. https://time.com/3556130/night-shift-brain-work-health/.

109. Panda, Satchin. *The Circadian Code.* (New York: Penguin Random House LLC, 2018), Pg. 6.

110. Ibid.

111. Ibid., Pg. 37.

112. Ibid.

113. Ibid., Pg. 40.

114. Ibid., Pg. 41.

115. De Cabo, Rafael & Matson, Mark. "Effects of Intermittent Fasting on Health, Aging, and Disease." *The New England Journal of Medicine Online*. December 26, 2019. Retrieved March 4, 2020. https://www.nejm.org/doi/full/10.1056/NEJMra1905136.

116. Kinouchi, Kenichiro; Magnan, Christophe; Ceglia, Nicholas, et. al. "Fasting Imparts a Switch to Alternative Daily Pathways in Liver and Muscle." *Cell Reports*. December 18, 2019. 3299-3314. Retrieved on March 4, 2020. https://www.cell.com/cell-reports/pdfExtended/S2211-1247(18)31868-0.

117. De Cabo & Matson, "Effects of Intermittent Fasting," Retrieved March 4, 2020.

118. Ibid.

119. Ibid.

120. English, Nick. "Autophagy: The Real Way to Cleanse Your Body. *Greatist Online*. July 1, 2019. Retrieved March 4, 2020. https://greatist.com/live/autophagy-fasting-exercise#definition.

121. Wu, Suzanne. "Fasting Triggers Stem Cell Regeneration of Damaged, Old Immune System." *USC News Online*. June 5, 2014. Retrieved April 24, 2020. https://news.usc.edu/63669/fasting-triggers-stem-cell-regeneration-of-damaged-old-immune-system/.

122. Jarreau, Paige. "The 5 Stages of Intermittent Fasting." *LifeApps Online*. February 26, 2019. Retrieved April 24, 2020. https://lifeapps.io/fasting/the-5-stages-of-intermittent-fasting/.

123. Ibid.

124. Ibid.

125. Ibid.

126. Ibid.

127. Ibid.

128. Ibid.

129. Ibid.

130. Ibid.

131. Ibid.

132. Wu, "Fasting Triggers," Retrieved April 24, 2020.

133. Jarreau, "The 5 Stages," Retrieved April 24, 2020.

134. Huang, Sabrina. "Fasting for 72 Hours Can Regenerate the Entire Immune System." *Six Senses Healing Online*. January 11, 2019. Retrieved April 24, 2020. https://www.sixsenseshealing.com/articles/2019/1/11/fasting-for-72-hours-can-regenerate-the-entire-immune-system.

135. Wu, "Fasting Triggers." Retrieved April 24, 2020.

136. Ibid.

137. Horn & Anderson, *Timebomb*. Pg. 210.

138. Arthur Wallis, *God's Chosen Fast*. (Christian Literature Crusade: Fort Washington, PA, 1968), Pg. 42.

139. Jarreau, "The 5 Stages." Retrieved April 24, 2020.

140. Ibid.

141. Gunnars, Kris. "Intermittent Fasting 101—The Ultimate Beginner's Guide." *Healthline Online*. April 20, 2020.Retrieved April 24, 2020. https://www.healthline.com/nutrition/intermittent-fasting-guide#methods.

142. Eugene, Andy & Masiak, Josh. "The Neuroprotective Aspects of Sleep." *US National Library of Medicine*. November 18, 2015. Retrieved March 4, 2020. https://www.ncbi.nlm.nih.gov/pmc/articles/PMC4651462/.

143. Roth, Thomas. "Slow Wave Sleep: Does It Matter?" *US National Library of Medicine*. April 15, 2009. Retrieved March 4, 2020. https://www.ncbi.nlm.nih.gov/pmc/articles/PMC2824210/.

144. Ibid.

145. "Restoring Deep, Slow Wave Sleep to Enhance Health and Increase Lifespan." *Nutrition Review*. July 5, 2014. Retrieved March 4, 2020. https://nutritionreview.org/2014/07/restoring-slow-wave-sleep-shown-enhance-health-increase-lifespan/.

146. Walker, Matthew. *Why We Sleep: Unlocking the Power of Sleep and Dreams.* (New York: Simon & Schuster), Pg. 27–28.

147. Ibid.

148. Ibid.

149. Ibid., Pg. 28–30.

150. "Why Electronics May Stimulate You Before Bed." *Sleep Foundation Online.* Retrieved march 4, 2020. https://www.sleepfoundation.org/articles/why-electronics-may-stimulate-you-bed.

151. Walker, *Why We Sleep,* Pg. 40.

152. "Understanding Sleep Cycles and the Stages of Sleep." *Whoop Online.* November 1, 2019. Retrieved March 4, 2020. https://www.whoop.com/the-locker/understanding-the-stages-of-sleep-how-to-optimize-it-with-whoop/.

153. "Restoring Deep, Slow Wave Sleep," *Nutrition Review.* Retrieved March 4, 2020.

154. "Sleep Longer to Lower Blood Glucose Levels." *Sleep Foundation Online.* Retrieved March 4, 2020. https://www.sleepfoundation.org/excessive-sleepiness/health-impact/sleep-longer-lower-blood-glucose-levels.

155. Ibid.

156. Ibid.

157. Hines, Jennifer. "Blood Sugar and Sleep Problems: How Blood Sugar Levels Impact Sleep." *Alaska Sleep Education Center Online.* August 7, 2018. Retrieved March 4, 2020. https://www.alaskasleep.com/blog/blood-sugar-and-sleep-problems.

158. Ibid.

159. Ibid.

160. Ibid.

161. "Restoring Deep, Slow Wave Sleep,"*Nutrition Review.* Retrieved March 4, 2020.

162. Hines, "Blood Sugar and Sleep Problems," Retrieved March 4, 2020.

163. "Restoring Deep, Slow Wave Sleep," *Nutrition Review.* Retrieved March 4, 2020.

164. Kuehn, Bridget. "Sleep Duration Linked to Cardiovascular Disease." *AHA Journals Online*. May 20, 2019. Retrieved March 5, 2020. https://www.ahajournals.org/doi/10.1161/CIRCULATIONAHA.119.041278.

165. Ibid.

166. Ibid.

167. Rettner, Rachel. "Here's How Poor Sleep May Hurt Your Heart." *Live Science Online*. February 13, 2019. Retrieved March 5, 2020. https://www.livescience.com/64761-sleep-heart-disease.html.

168. Ibid.

169. "Restoring Deep, Slow Wave Sleep," *Nutrition Review*, Retrieved March 4, 2020.

170. Andrew, Krystal. "Psychiatric Disorders and Sleep." *US National Library of Medicine*. November 30, 2012. Retrieved March 5, 2020. https://www.ncbi.nlm.nih.gov/pmc/articles/PMC3493205/.

171. Lo, June; Ong, Ju Lynn; Leong, Ruth, et. al. "Cognitive Performance, Sleepiness, and Mood in Partially Sleep Deprived Adolescents: The Need for Sleep Study." *Sleep Magazine, Vol. 39, Issue 3, p. 687-698*. March, 2016. Retrieved March 5, 2020. https://academic.oup.com/sleep/article/39/3/687/2454041.

172. Ibid.

173. Eugene & Masiak, , "Neuroprotective Aspects of Sleep," Retrieved March 4, 2020.

174. Walker, Matthew. "Cognitive Consequences of Sleep and Sleep Loss." *Science Direct Magazine, Vol. 9, Sup. 1, Pg. S29-S34*. Retrieved March 5, 2020. https://www.sciencedirect.com/science/article/abs/pii/S1389945708700145.

175. Mander, B. A., Rao, V., Lu, B., Saletin, J. M., Lindquist, J. R., Ancoli-israel, S., … Walker, M. P. (2013). Prefrontal atrophy, disrupted NREM slow waves and impaired hippocampal-dependent memory in aging. *Nature Neuroscience, 16*(3), 357–64. doi:http://dx.doi.org.ezproxy.regent.edu:2048/10.1038/nn.3324.

176. Ibid.

177. Walker, Matthew. "Sleep for Enhancing Learning, Creativity, Immunity, and Glymphatic System." *Found My Fitness*. February 28, 2019. Retrieved March 5, 2020. https://www.foundmyfitness.com/episodes/matthew-walker.

178. Ibid.

179. Ibid.

180. Ibid.

181. Ibid.

182. Ibid.

183. Ibid.

184. Ibid.

185. Ben Simon, E., & Walker, M. P. (2018). "Sleep Loss Causes Social Withdrawal and Loneliness." *Nature communications*, *9*(1), 3146. https://doi.org/10.1038/s41467-018-05377-0.

186. Ibid.

187. Adrian, Jonathan. "Why You've Been Sleeping All Wrong." *Medium Health*. September 14, 2019. Retrieved March 6, 2020. https://medium.com/@jonathanoei/why-youve-been-sleeping-all-wrong-87b2295314c0.

188. "Restoring Deep, Slow Wave Sleep." *Nutrition Review*. Retrieved March 4, 2020.

189. Ibid.

190. Ibid.

191. "Restoring Deep, Slow Wave." *Nutrition Review*. Retrieved March 4, 2020.

192. Zhang, Jun-Ming & An, Jianxiong. "Cytokines, Inflammation and Pain." *Us National Library of Medicine*. November 30, 2009. Retrieved March 6, 2020. https://www.ncbi.nlm.nih.gov/pmc/articles/PMC2785020/.

193. Ibid.

194. Ibid.

195. Ash, Michael. "Sleep and Its Detoxing Effect on the Brain and Body." *Clinical Education Online*. April 6, 2017. Retrieved March 6, 2020. https://www.clinicaleducation.org/news/sleep-and-its-detoxing-effect-on-the-brain-and-body/.

196. Roll. "GMOs, Glyphosate & Gut Health." Accessed January 8, 2020.

197. Ibid.

198. Kubala, Jillian. "7 Benefits and Uses of CBD Oil (Plus Side Effects)." *Healthline Online*. February 26, 2018. Retrieved March 11, 2020. https://www.healthline.com/nutrition/cbd-oil-benefits.

199. Ibid.

200. Alshamah, Asem. "What Is Nutrition?" *NutraHalal.* May 30, 2017. Retrieved March 6, 2020. http://www.nutra-halal.com/2017/05/30/what-is-nutrition/.

201. Ibid.

202. Roll, "Food Independence & Planetary Evolution," Retrieved March 6, 2020. https://www.youtube.com/watch?v=X3aOQ0N74PI.

203. "Malnutrition: Symptoms." *NHS Online*. February 7, 2020. Retrieved March 6, 2020. https://www.nhs.uk/conditions/malnutrition/symptoms/.

204. "What Are Macronutrients and Micronutrients?" *Natural Balanced Foods Online*. 2020. Retrieved March 6, 2020. https://www.naturalbalancefoods.com/community/dietary-needs/what-are-macronutrients-micronutrients/.

205. Ibid.

206. Osterweil, Neil. "The Benefits of Protein." *WebMD*. 2020. Retrieved March 6, 2020. https://www.webmd.com/men/features/benefits-protein#1.

207. "What Are Macronutrients and Micronutrients?" Retrieved March 6, 2020.

208. Cherney, Kristeen. "Simple Carbohydrates vs. Complex Carbohydrates." *Healthline Online*. December 18, 2018. Retrieved March 6, 2020. https://www.healthline.com/health/food-nutrition/simple-carbohydrates-complex-carbohydrates#simple-carbs.

209. Ibid.

210. "What Are Macronutrients and Micronutrients?" Retrieved March 6, 2020.

211. Healthline Editorial Team. "Nutritional Deficiencies (Malnutrition)." *Healthline Online*. February 13, 2018. https://www.healthline.com/nutrition/7-common-nutrient-deficiencies#section8.

212. Ibid.

213. Hjalmarsdottir, Freydis. "17 Science-Based Benefits of Omega-3 Fatty Acids." *Healthline Online.* October 15, 2018. Retrieved March 6, 2020. https://www.healthline.com/nutrition/17-health-benefits-of-omega-3.

214. Ibid.

215. Ibid.

216. Ibid.

217. Ibid.

218. Ibid.

219. Ibid.

220. "The Water in You: Water and the Human Body." *USGS Online.* 2020. Retrieved March 6, 2020. https://www.usgs.gov/special-topic/water-science-school/science/water-you-water-and-human-body?qt-science_center_objects=0#qt-science_center_objects.

221. Meletis, Chris. "Hydration & Electrolytes…It Takes More Than Just Water for Proper Hydration." *Trace Minerals Online.* 2020. Retrieved March 6, 2020. https://traceminerals.com/hydration-electrolytes-it-takes-more-than-just-water-for-proper-hydration/.

222. Bendix, Aria. "11 Terrifying Things That Could Be Lurking in Your Tap Water." *Business Insider.* July 5, 2019. Retrieved March 6, 2020. https://www.businessinsider.com/toxic-chemicals-tap-drinking-water-2019-4#mercury-from-industrial-waste-sites-can-pollute-well-water-11.

223. Ibid.

224. "Can Birth Control Hormones Be Filtered from the Water Supply?" *Scientific American Online.* July 28, 2009. Retrieved March 6, 2020. https://www.scientificamerican.com/article/birth-control-in-water-supply/.

225. "Can Birth Control Hormones Be Filtered?" Retrieved March 6, 2020.

226. Ibid.

227. Choi, Jean. "8 Awesome Benefits of Sea Salt." *What Great Grandma Ate Online.* May 15, 2017. Retrieved March 10, 2020. https://whatgreatgrandmaate.com/8-awesome-benefits-of-sea-salt/.

228. Ibid.

229. Ibid.

230. Lewin, Jo. "The Health Benefits of Fermenting." *BBC Good Food Online*. October 1, 2018. Retrieved March 10, 2020. https://www.bbcgoodfood. com/howto/guide/health-benefits-offermenting.

231. Ibid.

232. Ibid.

233. "Gut Microbiota of Infants Predicts Obesity in Children." *Science News Online*. October 23, 2018. Retrieved March 10, 2020. https://www. sciencedaily.com/releases/2018/10/181023085640.htm.

234. "Ibid.

235. "The Brain-Gut Connection." *Hopkins Medicine Online*. 2020. Retrieved March 10, 2020. https://www.hopkinsmedicine.org/health/ wellness-and-prevention/the-brain-gut-connection.

236. Ibid.

237. Ibid.

238. Ibid.

239. "Gut Bacteria May Play a Role in Alzheimer's Disease." *Neurodegeneration Research Online*. April 6, 2017. https://www.neurodegenerationresearch. eu/2017/04/gut-bacteria-may-play-a-role-in-alzheimers-disease/.

240. Perez-Pardo, Paula; Kliest, Tessa; & Dodiya, Hemraj; et. al. "The Gut-Brain Axis in Parkinson's Disease: Possibilities for Food-Based Therapies." *European Journal of Pharmacology*, Vol. 817, p. 86–95. December 15, 2017. Retrieved March 10, 2020. https://www.sciencedirect.com/science/ article/pii/S0014299917303734.

241. "The Gut-Brain Connection." *Harvard Health Publishing Online*. 2020. Retrieved March 10, 2020. https://www.health.harvard.edu/ diseases-and-conditions/the-gut-brain-connection.

242. "4 Tips for a Happier Gut and a Healthier You." *AP News Online*. March 20, 2019. Retrieved March 10, 2020. https://apnews.com/a18e644abb99 4b3ca76211179751129b.

243. Hyman, Mark. "How Good Gut Health Can Boost Your Immune System." *EcoWatch Online*. February 26, 2015. Retrieved March 10,

2020. https://www.ecowatch.com/how-good-gut-health-can-boost-your-immune-system-1882013643.html.

244. Bodian, C. H. "4 Positive Effects of Exercise on the Digestive System." *Livestrong Online.* March 8, 2019. Retrieved March 10, 2020. https://www.livestrong.com/article/356356-immediate-effects-of-exercise-in-the-digestive-system/.

245. Ibid.

246. Robinson, Jo. "Breeding the Nutrition Out of Our Food." *The New York Times,* 25 May 2013, http://www.nytimes.com/2013/05/26/opinion/sunday/breeding-the-nutrition-out-of-our-food.html?pagewanted=all. Accessed 18 Dec. 2017.

247. Sarrasin, Shannon. "10 Benefits of Digestive Bitters." *Lifestyle Markets Online.* February 23, 2017. Retrieved March 10, 2020. https://lifestylemarkets.com/blog/10-benefits-of-digestive-bitters/.

248. Horn & Anderson, *Timebomb,* Pg. 126.

249. "The Importance of Chewing Your Food." *Heritage Integrative Healthcare Online.* 2020. Retrieved March 10, 2020. http://heritageihc.com/blog/chewing-your-food/.

250. "What Is Methylation and Why Should You Care?" *Revolution Health & Wellness Online.* 2020. Retrieved March 10, 2020. https://www.revolutionhealth.org/what-is-methylation-and-why-should-you-care/.

251. Ibid.

252. Ibid.

253. Ibid.

254. Marcin, Ashley. "What You Need to Know About the MTHFR Gene." *Healthline Online.* August 14, 2019. https://www.healthline.com/health/mthfr-gene#testing.

255. "What Is Methylation and Why Should You Care?" Retrieved March 10, 2020.

256. Marcin, Ashley. "What You Need to Know," August 14, 2019.

257. Ibid.

258. Ibid.

259. "What Are Single Nucleotide Polymorphisms (SNPs)?" U.S. National Library of Medicine Online. 2020. Retrieved April 24, 2020. https://ghr.nlm.nih.gov/primer/genomicresearch/snp.

260. "Body System Communication." Victoria State Government: Education and Training. November, 2018. Retrieved April 24, 2020. https://www.education.vic.gov.au/school/teachers/teachingresources/discipline/science/continuum/Pages/bodysysteb.aspx.

261. Ibid.

262. Grimm, Jana. "MTHF-R Gene Mutation: 50% of Americans & 95% of Autistic people." *Dr. Jana Joshu Grimm, DC Wellness Blog Online.* May 17, 2017. Retrieved April 24, 2020. https://www.drjanajoshugrimm.com/wellness-blog/mthfr-gene-mutation-50-of-americans-95-of-autistic-people.

263. Mayo Clinic. "Many Benefits of Exercise: Mayo Clinic Radio." April 25, 2018. Facebook Watch Online. Retrieved from https://www.facebook.com/watch/?v=10155400852532517.

264. Jaslow, Ryan. "CDC: 80 Percent of American Adults Don't Get Recommended Exercise." *CBS News Online.* May 3, 2013. Retrieved March 10, 2020. https://www.cbsnews.com/news/cdc-80-percent-of-american-adults-dont-get-recommended-exercise/.

265. Poon, Linda. "The Rise and Fall of New Year's Fitness Resolutions, in 5 Charts." *City Lab Online.* January 16, 2019. Retrieved March 10, 2020. https://www.citylab.com/life/2019/01/do-people-keep-new-years-resolution-fitness-weight-loss-data/579388/.

266. Van Hare, Holly. "The Real Reason You Hate Working Out, According to Science." *The Active Times Online.* February 25, 2019. Retrieved March 10, 2020. https://www.theactivetimes.com/fitness/why-hate-working-out-science.

267. Ibid.

268. Steinhilber, Brianna. "The Health Benefits of Working Out with a Crowd." *NBC News Online.* September 15, 2017. Retrieved March 10, 2020. https://www.nbcnews.com/better/health/why-you-should-work-out-crowd-ncna798936.

269. Ibid.
270. Wing, R. R., & Jeffery, R. W. (1999). "Benefits of Recruiting Participants with Friends and Increasing Social Support for Weight Loss and Maintenance." *Journal of Consulting and Clinical Psychology*, 67(1), 132–138. https://doi.org/10.1037/0022-006X.67.1.132.
271. Ibid.
272. "Vagus Nerve." *Encyclopedia Britannica*. 2020. Retrieved April 27, 2020. https://www.britannica.com/science/vagus-nerve.
273. Foxo Health. "How to Stay Young with Mitochondrial Biogenesis." March 6, 2020. YouTube Video, 9:05. Retrieved March 10, 2020. https://www.youtube.com/watch?v=AefLdrQ8s1k.
274. Ibid.
275. Macmillan, Amanda. "Exercise Makes You Younger at the Cellular Level." *Time Magazine Online*. May 15, 2017. Retrieved March 10, 2020. https://time.com/4776345/exercise-aging-telomeres/.
276. Ibid.
277. Salk Institute. "Satchin Panda—Circadian Theory of Health." September 13, 2018. YouTube Video, 55:07. Retrieved March 10, 2020. https://www.youtube.com/watch?v=LJ9Ae_j_kjI.
278. Ibid.
279. Roll, "GMOs, Glyphosate & Gut Health." Accessed January 8, 2020.
280. Joanisse, Sophie; Snijders, Tim; Neverdeen, Joshua; et. al. "The Impact of Aerobic Exercise on the Muscle Stem Cell Response." *Exercise and Sport Sciences Reviews Online*. July 2018, Vol. 46, Issue 3, p. 180-187. Retrieved March 10, 2020. https://journals.lww.com/acsm-essr/Fulltext/2018/07000/The_Impact_of_Aerobic_Exercise_on_the_Muscle_Stem.7.aspx.
281. Ibid.
282. Ibid.
283. Mayo Clinic. "Many Benefits of Exercise: Mayo Clinic Radio." April 25, 2018. Facebook Watch Online. Retrieved from https://www.facebook.com/watch/?v=10155400852532517.

284. Ibid.

285. Riske, Laurel; Rejish, Thomas; Baker, Glen; et. al. *US National Library of Medicine Online*. October 28, 2016. Retrieved March 10, 2020. https://www.ncbi.nlm.nih.gov/pmc/articles/PMC5315230/.

286. University of Zurich. "Lactate for Brain Energy." November 24, 2015. Retrieved March 10, 2020. https://www.sciencedaily.com/releases/2015/11/151124082233.htm.

287. Lev-Vachnish, Yaeli; Cadury, Sharon; Rotter-Maskowitz, Aviva; et. al. "l-Lactate Promotes Adult Hippocampal Neurogenesis." *US National Library of Medicine*. May 24, 2019. Retrieved March 10, 2020. https://www.ncbi.nlm.nih.gov/pmc/articles/PMC6542996/.

288. Godman, Heidi. "Regular Exercise Changes the Brain to Improve Memory, Thinking Skills." *Harvard Health Magazine Online*. April 9, 2014. Retrieved March 10, 2020. https://www.health.harvard.edu/blog/regular-exercise-changes-brain-improve-memory-thinking-skills-201404097110.

289. Hearing, C. M.; Chang, W. C.; Szuhanay, K. L.; et. al. "Physical Exercise for Treatment of Mood Disorders: A Critical Review." *US National Library of Medicine*. October 14, 2016. Retrieved March 10, 2020. https://www.ncbi.nlm.nih.gov/pmc/articles/PMC5423723/.

290. Ibid.

291. Collins, Ryan. "Exercise, Depression, and the Brain." *Healthline Online*. March 29, 2016. Retrieved March 10, 2020. https://www.healthline.com/health/depression/exercise#1.

292. Hearing, Chang, Szuhanay, et. Al, "Physical Exercise" Retrieved March 10, 2020.

293. Collins, Ryan. "Exercise, Depression, and the Brain." Retrieved March 10, 2020.

294. "More Evidence That Exercise Can Boost Mood." *Harvard Health Publishing Online*. May 2019. Retrieved March 10, 2020. https://www.health.harvard.edu/mind-and-mood/more-evidence-that-exercise-can-boost-mood.

295. "The Many Ways Exercise Helps Your Heart." *Harvard Health Magazine Online*. March 2018. Retrieved March 10, 2020. https://www.health. harvard.edu/heart-health/the-many-ways-exercise-helps-your-heart.

296. Ibid.

297. Pinckard, Kelsey; Baskin, Kedryn; & Stanford, Kristin. "Effects of Exercise to Improve Cardiovascular Health." *Frontiers in Cardiovascular Medicine*. June 4, 2019. Retrieved March 10, 2020. https://www.frontiersin.org/ articles/10.3389/fcvm.2019.00069/full.

298. Sheff, Breathe. 'Your Lungs and Exercise." *US National Library of Medicine*. March 12, 2016. Retrieved March 10, 2020. https://www.ncbi. nlm.nih.gov/pmc/articles/PMC4818249/.

299. "Exercise and Lung Health." *American Lung Association*. 2020. Retrieved March 10, 2020. https://www.lung.org/lung-health-and-diseases/ protecting-your-lungs/exercise-and-lung-health.html.

300. "Exercising for Better Sleep." *Hopkins Medicine Online*. 2020. Retrieved March 10, 2020. https://www.hopkinsmedicine.org/health/ wellness-and-prevention/exercising-for-better-sleep.

301. Ibid.

302. Peloquin, Andrew. "How Exercise Affects Your Metabolism." 2020. Retrieved March 10, 2020. https://www.fitday.com/fitness-articles/fitness/ how-exercise-affects-your-metabolism.html.

303. Ibid.

304. Ibid.

305. Cohut, Maria. "How Exercise Tells the Brain to Curb Appetite." *Medical News Today*. April 29, 2018. Retrieved March 10, 2020. https://www. medicalnewstoday.com/articles/321660#Neural-receptors-regulate-feeding.

306. Ibid.

307. American Physiological Society. "Exercise Suppresses Appetite by Affecting Appetite Hormones." December 19, 2008. Retrieved March 10, 2020. https://www.sciencedaily.com/releases/2008/12/081211081446.htm.

308. Ibid.

309. "George Bernard Shaw Quotes." *Brainy Quote Online*. 2020.

Retrieved March 10, 2020. https://www.brainyquote.com/quotes/george_bernard_shaw_120971.

310. "The Role of Vitamin D in Digestive Health." Rocky Mountain Analytical. April 5, 2018. http://www.rmalab.com/role-vitamin-d-digestive-health.

311. Spritzler, Franziska. "8 Signs and Symptoms of Vitamin D Deficiency." *Healthline Online.* July 23, 2018. https://www.healthline.com/nutrition/vitamin-d-deficiency-symptoms.

312. "Late-night Eating and Melatonin May Impair Insulin Response." *Found My Fitness Online.* April 2, 2019. Retrieved March 10, 2020. https://www.foundmyfitness.com/episodes/melatonin-insulin-response.

313. Ibid.

314. Spritzler, Franziska. "8 Signs and Symptoms of Vitamin D Deficiency." July 23, 2018.

315. Forrest, K. Y. & Stuhldreher, W. L. "Prevalence and Correlates of Vitamin D Deficiency in US Adults. *US National Library of Medicine.* January 31, 2011. Retrieved March 10, 2020. https://www.ncbi.nlm.nih.gov/pubmed/21310306.

316. Jacobsen, Rowan. "Is Sunscreen the New Margarine?" *Outside Online.* January 10, 2019. Retrieved March 10, 2020. https://www.outsideonline.com/2380751/sunscreen-sun-exposure-skin-cancer-science.

317. Jat, K. R. "Vitamin D Deficiency and Lower Respiratory Tract Infections in Children: A systematic Review and Meta-analysis of Observational Studies." *US National Library of Medicine.* Epub May 13, 2016. Retrieved March 10, 2020. https://www.ncbi.nlm.nih.gov/pubmed/27178217.

318. Zhang, Jun-Ming & An, Jianxiong. "Cytokines, Inflammation and Pain." *US National Library of Medicine.* November 30, 2009. Retrieved March 10, 2020. https://www.ncbi.nlm.nih.gov/pmc/articles/PMC2785020/.

319. Ghai, B.; Bansal, D.; & Kapil, G. et. al. "High Prevalence of Hypovitaminosis D in Indian Chronic Low Back Patients." *US National Library of Medicine.* October 18, 2015. Retrieved March 10, 2020. https://www.ncbi.nlm.nih.gov/pubmed/26431139.

320. Erkal, M. Z.; Wilde, J.; & Bilgin, Y. et. al. "High Prevalence of Vitamin D Deficiency, Secondary Hyperparathyroidism and Generalized Bone Pain in Turkish Immigrants in Germany: Identification of Risk Factors." *US National Library of Medicine.* Epub May 23, 2006. Retrieved March 10, 2020. https://www.ncbi.nlm.nih.gov/pubmed/16718398.

321. "Secondary Hyperparathyroidism." *Columbia University Irving Medical Center Online.* 2020. Retrieved March 10, 2020. https://columbiasurgery. org/conditions-and-treatments/secondary-hyperparathyroidism.

322. Erkal, Wilde, & Bilgin, et. al. "High Prevalence of Vitamin D deficiency," Retrieved March 10, 2020..

323. Talaei, Afsaneh; Ghorbani, Fariba; & Asemi, Zatollah. "The Effects of Vitamin D Supplementation on Thyroid Function in Hypothyroid Patients: A Randomized, Double-blind, Placebo-controlled Trial." *US National Library of Medicine: Indian J Endocrinol Metab., V 22, Issue 5, p. 584-588.* September/October 2018. Retrieved March 10, 2020. https:// www.ncbi.nlm.nih.gov/pmc/articles/PMC6166548/.

324. Bener, A. & Saleh, N. M. "Low Vitamin D, and Bone Mineral Density with Depressive Symptoms Burden in Menopausal and Postmenopausal Women." *J Midlife Health, July-September; 6 (3) 108-14. As cited by US National Library of Medicine.* Retrieved March 10, 2020. https://www. ncbi.nlm.nih.gov/pubmed/26538987.

325. Kostoglou-Athanassiou, Ifigenia; Athanassiou, Panagiotis; & Lyraki, Aikaterini; et. al. "Vitamin D and Rheumatoid Arthritis." *Ther Adv Endocrinol Metab, Vol. 3, Issue 6, p. 181–187.* December 2012. As cited by *US National Library of Medicine.* Retrieved March 10, 2020. https://www. ncbi.nlm.nih.gov/pmc/articles/PMC3539179/.

326. "State Statistics: State-Specific 2015 BRFSS Arthritis Prevalence Estimates." *CDC Online.* July 18, 2018. Retrieved March 10, 2020. https://www.cdc.gov/arthritis/data_statistics/state-data-current.htm.

327. "Average Annual Sunshine by State." *Current Results Online.* 2020. Retrieved March 10, 2020. https://www.currentresults.com/Weather/US/ average-annual-state-sunshine.php.

328. "State Statistics: State-Specific 2015 BRFSS Arthritis Prevalence Estimates." *CDC Online*. July 18, 2018. Retrieved March 10, 2020. https://www.cdc.gov/arthritis/data_statistics/state-data-current.htm.

329. Garland, Cedric; Garland, Frank; & Gorham, Edward; et. al. "The Role of Vitamin D in Cancer Prevention." *American Journal of Public Health, Vol. 96, Issue 2*, p. 252–261. As cited by *US National Library of Medicine*. February 2006. Retrieved March 10, 2020. https://www.ncbi.nlm.nih.gov/pmc/articles/PMC1470481/.

330. Ibid.

331. Ibid.

332. Garland, Cedric & Garland, Frank. "Do Sunlight and Vitamin D Reduce the Likelihood of Colon Cancer?" *Oxford Academic Online*. November 22, 2005. Retrieved March 10, 2020. https://academic.oup.com/ije/article/35/2/217/694653.

333. Ibid.

334. Carey, Benedict & Gebeloff, Robert. "Many People Taking Antidepressants Discover They Cannot Quit." *New York Times* as cited on *Pharmacist Online*. April 7, 2018. Retrieved March 10, 2020. https://www.pharmacist.com/article/many-people-taking-antidepressants-discover-they-cannot-quit.

335. Ibid.

336. Jorde, R.; Sneve, M.; & Figenschau, Y.; et. al. "Effects of Vitamin D Supplementation on Symptoms of Depression in Overweight and Obese Subjects: Randomized Double Blind Trial." *J Intern Med, Vol. 264, Issue 6*. As cited on *US National Library of Medicine*. December 2008. Retrieved March 10, 2020. https://www.ncbi.nlm.nih.gov/pubmed/18793245.

337. Okereke, O. & Singh, A. "The Role of Vitamin D in the Prevention of Late-Life Depression." *J Affect Disord, Epub* as cited by *US National Library of Medicine*. March 9, 2016. Retrieved March 10, 2020. https://www.ncbi.nlm.nih.gov/pubmed/26998791.

338. Robinson, S. L.; Marin, C.; & Oliveros, H. et. al. *J Nutr Vol. 150, Issue 1*, Pg. 140–148. As cited by *US National Library of Medicine*. January

2020. Retrieved March 10, 2020. https://www.ncbi.nlm.nih.gov/pubmed/31429909.

339. "Seasonal Affective Disorder (SAD)." *Mayo Clinic Online.* 2020. Retrieved March 10, 2020. https://www.mayoclinic.org/diseases-conditions/seasonal-affective-disorder/symptoms-causes/syc-20364651.

340. "Seasonal Affective Disorder." *Psychology Today.* 2020. Retrieved March 10, 2020. https://www.psychologytoday.com/us/conditions/seasonal-affective-disorder.

341. "Sunshine for SAD Sufferers." *Web MD.* 2020. Retrieved March 10, 2020. https://www.webmd.com/depression/features/sunshine-for-sad-sufferers#1.

342. Labban, Louay. "Seasonal Affective Disorder (SAD), Vitamin D Deficiency and Diabetes Mellitus." *Science Open Access Online.* August 11, 2017. Retrieved March 10, 2020. https://scientonline.org/open-access/seasonal-affective-disorder-sad-vitamin-d-deficiency-and-diabetes-mellitus.pdf.

343. Miller, Craig. "Seasonal Affective Disorder: Bring on the Light." *Harvard Health Magazine Online.* October 29, 2015. Retrieved March 10, 2020. https://www.health.harvard.edu/blog/seasonal-affective-disorder-bring-on-the-light-201212215663.

344. Ibid.

345. "Sunshine for SAD Sufferers." Retrieved March 10, 2020. .

346. Schmidt, Sigrun; Ording, Anne; & Horvath-Puho, Erzsebet. "Non-melanoma Skin Cancer and Risk of Alzheimer's Disease and All-Cause Dementia." *US National Library of Medicine.* February 22, 2017. Retrieved March 10, 2020. https://www.ncbi.nlm.nih.gov/pmc/articles/PMC5321271/.

347. Weller, R. B. "Sunlight Has Cardiovascular Benefits Independently of Vitamin D." *Karger Online.*2016. Retrieved March 1, 2020. https://www.karger.com/Article/FullText/441266.

348. Paddock, Catharine. "Vitamin D-3 Could 'Reverse' Damage to Heart." *Medical News Today Online.* February 1, 2018. Retrieved March 11, 2020. https://www.medicalnewstoday.com/articles/320802.

349. Ibid.

350. Ibid.

351. Grimes, D. S.; Hindle, E. & Dyer, T. "Sunlight, Cholesterol and Coronary Heart Disease." *QJ Med, Vol. 89;* as available through Oxford University Press. May 9, 1996. p. 579–589.

352. Ibid.

353. Ibid.

354. Ibid.

355. Paddock, Catharine. "Vitamin D-3," Retrieved March 11, 2020.

356. Raman, Ryan. "How to Safely Get Vitamin D from Sunlight." *Healthline Online.* April 28, 2018. Retrieved April 27, 2020. https://www.healthline.com/nutrition/vitamin-d-from-sun#dangers.

357. Ibid.

358. Zolfagharifard, Ellie. "Do You Have EMAIL APNOEA? 80% of People Stop Breathing Properly When Typing——And It Could Be Damaging Our Health." *Daily Mail Online.* November 18, 2013. Retrieved March 11, 2020. https://www.dailymail.co.uk/sciencetech/article-2509391/Do-EMAIL-APNOEA-80-people-stop-breathing-properly-typing.html.

359. Ibid.

360. Lawrence, Gwen. "Breathing Is Believing: The Importance of Nasal Breathing." *GAIAM Online.* 2020. Retrieved March 11, 2020. https://www.gaiam.com/blogs/discover/breathing-is-believing-the-importance-of-nasal-breathing.

361. Ibid.

362. Ibid.

363. "Benefits of Oxygen." *Valeo Wellness Center Online.* 2020. Retrieved March 11, 2020. https://valeowc.com/services/neurometabolic/benefits-of-oxygen/.

364. Lawrence, Gwen. "Breathing Is Believing," Retrieved March 11, 2020.

365. Ibid.

366. Ibid.

367. Davis, Charles. "Hypoxia and Hypoxemia." *Medicine Net.* 2020.

Retrieved March 11, 2020. https://www.medicinenet.com/hypoxia_and_hypoxemia/article.htm.

368. Norman, Muhammad; Hasmim, Meriem; & Messai, Yosra; et. al. *American Journal Physiol Cell Physiol. Vol. 309, Issue 9, C 569–579. As cited by US National Library of Medicine*. November 1, 2015. Retrieved March 11, 2020. https://www.ncbi.nlm.nih.gov/pmc/articles/PMC4628936/.

369. "Oxygen Can Impair Cancer Immunotherapy in Mice." *National Institutes of Health Online*. August 25, 2016. Retrieved March 11, 2020. https://www.nih.gov/news-events/news-releases/oxygen-can-impair-cancer-immunotherapy-mice.

370. Ibid.

371. Ibid.

372. "Oxygen plays a pivotal role in the proper functioning of the immune e system. We can look at oxygen deficiency as the single greatest cause of all diseases." *Quotefancy Online*. 2020. Retrieved March 11, 2020. https://quotefancy.com/quote/1516986/Stephen-Levine-Oxygen-plays-a-pivotal-role-in-the-proper-functioning-of-the-immune-system.

373. Clavel, Alfred. "Why Opioids Make Pain Worse." *Health Partners Online*. 2020. Retrieved March 11, 2020. https://www.healthpartners.com/blog/why-opioids-make-pain-worse/.

374. Ibid.

375. "Caution: These Are the Most Addictive Pain Meds." *Harvard Health Publishing Online*. November, 2013. Retrieved March 11, 2020. https://www.health.harvard.edu/diseases-and-conditions/caution-these-are-the-most-addictive-pain-meds.

376. Sinay, Danielle. "Is Acupuncture the Miracle Remedy for Everything?" *Healthline Online*. November 30, 2017. Retrieved March 11, 2020. https://www.healthline.com/health/acupuncture-how-does-it-work-scientifically#how-does-it-work.

377. Sinay, Danielle. "Is Acupuncture the Miracle Remedy for Everything?" *Healthline Online*. November 30, 2017. Retrieved March 11, 2020. https://www.healthline.com/health/acupuncture-how-does-it-work-scientifically#how-does-it-work.

378. Ibid.

379. Kubala, Jillian. "7 Benefits and Uses of CBD Oil (Plus Side Effects)." *Healthline Online.* February 26, 2018. Retrieved March 11, 2020. https://www.healthline.com/nutrition/cbd-oil-benefits.

380. Ibid.

381. Iseger, T. A. & Bossong, M. G. "A Systematic Review of the Antipsychotic Properties of Cannabidiol in Humans." Schizophr Res. Vol. 162, Issue 1–3, Epub. As cited by US National Library of Medicine. February 2015. Retrieved March 11, 2020. https://www.ncbi.nlm.nih.gov/pubmed/25667194.

382. Kubala, Jillian. "7 Benefits," Retrieved March 11, 2020.

383. Jadoon, Khalid; Tan, Garry; & O'Sullivan, Saoirse. "A Single Dose of Cannabidiol Reduces Blood Pressure in Healthy Volunteers in a Randomized Study." *JCI Insight, as cited by US National Library of Medicine.* June 15, 2017. Retrieved March 11, 2020. https://www.ncbi.nlm.nih.gov/pmc/articles/PMC5470879/.

384. Devinsky, O.; Cross, J. H.; & Laux, L. et. al. "Trial of Cannabidiol for Drug-Resistant Seizures in the Dravet Syndrome." *New England Journal of Medicine, as cited by US National Library of Medicine.* May 25, 2017. Retrieved March 11, 2020. https://www.ncbi.nlm.nih.gov/pubmed/28538134.

385. Prud'homme, Melissa; Cata, Romulus; & Jutras-Aswad, Didier. "Cannabidiol as an Intervention for Addictive Behaviors: A Systematic Review of the Evidence." *Subst. Abuse, as cited by US National Library of Medicine.* May 21, 2015. Retrieved March 11, 2020. https://www.ncbi.nlm.nih.gov/pmc/articles/PMC4444130/.

386. Weiss, L.; Zeira, M. & Reich, S. et. al. "Cannabidiol Lowers Incidence of Diabetes in Non-obese Diabetic Mice." *Autoimmunity, as cited by US National Library of Medicine.* March, 2006. Retrieved March 11, 2020. https://www.ncbi.nlm.nih.gov/pubmed/16698671.

387. Shrivastava, A.; Kuzontkoski, P.M.; & Groopman, J.E. et. al. "Cannabidiol Induces Programmed Cell Death in Breast Cancer Cells by Coordinating the Cross-talk Between Apoptosis and Autophagy." *Mol Cancer Ther. Vol.*

     10, Issue 7, pg. 1161–1172, as cited by US National Library of Medicine. July, 2011. Retrieved March 11, 2020. https://www.ncbi.nlm.nih.gov/pubmed/21566064.

388. McAllister, S.D.; Soroceanu, L.; & Desprez, P.Y. "The Antitumor Activity of Plant-Derived Non-Psychoactive Cannabinoids." *J Neuroimmune Pharmacol., Epub. As cited by US National Library of Medicine.* June 2015. Retrieved March 11, 2020. https://www.ncbi.nlm.nih.gov/pubmed/25916739.

389. Clavel, Alfred. "Why Opioids Make Pain Worse." *Health Partners Online.* 2020. Retrieved March 11, 2020. https://www.healthpartners.com/blog/why-opioids-make-pain-worse/.

390. Roland, James. "Is E-Stim the Answer to Your Pain?" *Healthline Online.* July 29, 2019. Retrieved March 11, 2020. https://www.healthline.com/health/pain-relief/e-stim.

391. Caceres, Vanessa & Schroeder, Michael. "What's Driving the Rise in Type 2 Diabetes in Kids?" *U.S. News Health Online.* April 9, 2019. Retrieved April 27, 2020. https://health.usnews.com/health-care/patient-advice/articles/2017-07-25/why-type-2-diabetes-is-on-the-rise-in-children-and-teens.